GROUP PSYCHOTHERAPIES FOR
THE ELDERLY

GROUP PSYCHOTHERAPIES FOR THE ELDERLY

edited by

BERYCE W. MACLENNAN, Ph.D.,

SHURA SAUL, Ed.D., B.C.C.S.W.,

and

MARCELLA BAKUR WEINER, Ed.D.

with the assistance of

JUNE E. BLUM, Ph.D.,

MAURICE LINDEN, M.D.,

and

JACK SKIGEN, M.D.

Monograph 5

AMERICAN GROUP PSYCHOTHERAPY ASSOCIATION
MONOGRAPH SERIES

Series Consulting Editor:
Walter N. Stone, M.D.

INTERNATIONAL UNIVERSITIES PRESS, INC.
Madison   Connecticut

Library of Congress Cataloging-in-Publication Data

Group psychotherapies for the elderly.

(Monograph series/American Group Psychotherapy Association; monograph 5)
   Includes bibliographies and index.
   1. Geriatric psychiatry.   2. Group psychotherapy.
I. MacLennan, Beryce W.   II. Saul, Shura.   III. Weiner,
Marcella Bakur, 1925–   .   IV. Series: Monograph
series (American Group Psychotherapy Association;
monograph 5. [DNLM: 1. Psychotherapy, Group — in old age.
W1 M0559PU monograph 5/WT 150 G882]
RC451.4.A5G76   1988   618.97' 689152   87-35297
ISBN 0-8236-2252-5

Manufactured in the United States of America.

This monograph is dedicated to the memory of Maurice Linden, M.D., one of AGPA's early presidents and a pioneer in the use of group therapy with elderly mental patients. But for his illness and death in 1984, personal reminiscences of his early experiences would have been included in this monograph. We all miss his knowledge and skill and his sympathetic understanding.

Contents

Contributors

Aronson, Miriam K.
Assistant Professor Neurology & Psychiatry, Albert Einstein College of Medicine, Bronx, New York

Benitez Bloch, Rosalyn, D.S.W.
Supervisor Airport Marina Counseling Center, Los Angeles, California

Bienenfeld, David, M.D.
Director, Division of Geropsychiatry, University of Cincinnati Medical Center, Cincinnati, Ohio

Blum, June, Ph.D.
Clinical Assistant Professor, Psychology, Cornell University Medical College, New York City

Fisher, Daniel B., M.D., Ph.D.
Psychiatric Director, Eastern Middlesex Area, Department of Human Services, Wakefield, Massachusetts

Goodman, Ruth K., M.S.W., Director Emeritus (Rtd)
Department of Social Work, Payne Whitney Clinic, New York Hospital, New York City

Hainer, Jeanette, A.C.S.W.
Director Senior Adult Division, 92nd Street Y, New York City

Lakin, Martin, Ph.D.
Professor, Department of Psychology, Duke University, Durham, North Carolina

Lothstein, Leslie M., Ph.D.
Director, Department of Clinical Psychology, The Institute for Living, Hartford, Connecticut

MacLennan, Beryce W., Ph.D.
Professor, Department of Medicine and Behavioral Science, George Washington University, Washington, D.C.

Moerman, Constance, M.A.
Professor, Psychology, Montgomery County College, Takoma Park, Maryland

Matorin, Susan, B.C.S.W.
Director, Department of Social Work, Payne Whitney Clinic, New York Hospital, New York City

Morrin, Jane, M.A.
> Art Therapist, Private Practice, New York City

Rathbone-McCuan, Eloise, Ph.D.
> C.S.W. Director, Social Work, University of Vermont, Burlington, Vermont

Schloss, Gilbert A., Ph.D.
> C.S.W. Institute of Sociotherapy, New York City

Saul, Shura, Ed.D., B.C.S.W.
> Educational Coordinator, Kingsbridge Heights Manor (rtd) and Adjunct Professor, Yeshiva University, New York

Saul, Sidney, Ed.D., B.C.S.W.
> Psychogeriatric Consultant, New York City

Skigen, Jack, M.D.
> Chief Medical Officer, Miami Jewish Home and Hospital, Miami, Florida

Stern, Ronica, Ed.M., M.A.
> Drama Gerontologist, Private Practice, Berkeley, California

Samberg, Sonya, G.D.T.
> Movement Specialist and Consultant to geriatric institutions in New York City

Tross, Susan, Ph.D.
> Lecturer, Psychology, Department of Psychiatry, Cornell University Medical School, New York City

Weiner, Marcella B., Ed.D.
> Adjunct Professor, Brooklyn College

Weiner, William, C.S.W.
> Veterans Administration Hospital, Bronx, New York

White, Marjorie Taggart, Ph.D.
> Member, Faculty & Advisory Council, American Institute for Psychotherapy and Psychoanalysis, New York

Zoubok, Boris
> Director, Neuropsychiatric Evaluation, Four Winds Hospital, Valhalla, New York

Introduction

BERYCE W. MACLENNAN, Ph.D.

One of the most striking demographic trends noted in recent years is a dramatic and continuing expansion in the number of older people. In 1980 there were twenty-six million elderly living in the United States. By 2030, it is projected, that figure will reach fifty million.

The vast majority of people over sixty-five are active, reasonably healthy, and mentally alert. However, our society creates problems for this population, as it has not yet accommodated to the idea of so many active, competent people living long into their sixties, seventies, and eighties, and even into their nineties and beyond. Consequently, many younger and more active elderly need assistance in reassessing their prospects for their later years and in maintaining a satisfactory adjustment to old age. Furthermore, the number of elderly over eighty is increasing even more rapidly than the young elderly population, and a much higher proportion of the former suffer chronic physical and mental handicaps. We need to improve our methods of treating these handicapped elderly who may live ten or twenty years beyond the age of eighty.

Although there is a continuum of condition and need experienced by the young active elderly and the older, frail elderly, there are major differences between older people who see themselves as still functioning in the adult world and those who are coping with a range of disabilities that may include disorientation and confusion. Mental health professionals, attracted by the increased demand for service, are entering the field of psychosocial geriatrics and are trying out many different methods of group therapy for the elderly and their relatives. We may ask, why group therapy? Group therapy is often the treatment of choice because groups encourage the identification of common problems and the examination of diverse solutions; they reduce the shame of having mental health problems and render them more socially acceptable. Groups provide opportunities for mutual caring, enhance self-esteem, and reduce social isolation and loneliness, common problems among the elderly.

Many different forms of group therapy, psychotherapy, counseling, behavior modification, and activity therapy are being tried with the elderly. Some of the young elderly face barriers in their careers or the loss of friends and relatives; they may also have to deal with their own elderly parents. These individuals may prefer treatment in a group of people who are heterogeneous in age and who are struggling with a wide variety of intrapsychic and interpersonal problems. Others, in similar situations, find it more useful to come together with peers to examine situational crises experienced in common. Some older adults, while still physically and mentally capable, experience deep depression due to changes in self-image, reductions in intimacy and social life, or from developing biological dysfunctions. Ingenuity may be required to identify and reach out to these people, who tend to stay isolated in their homes but who can benefit greatly from group therapy.

Groups for the more disabled elderly are often developed in more specialized settings: retirement homes, centers for the aging, nursing homes, hospitals. These groups are sometimes integrated into activities such as art, music, poetry, or drama. These provide the stimulation critical in maintaining ego identity and integrity in the frail elderly.

Relatives of the elderly experience many stresses in arranging their lives to sustain those dear to them who are deteriorating physically and mentally. Psychic pain is often compounded by material difficulties, and support groups can be very helpful in providing encouragement as well as information about resources.

Mental health professionals and other care providers working with the elderly find that they must deal not only with their patients' biases and stereotypes about aging but also with their own. They may find themselves unwilling to face their own anxieties regarding disability and death. Underestimating the rich resources found in any group of elderly they may unduly foster dependency. Groups focused on these issues may increase the self-awareness of those planning to work with the elderly.

This monograph examines a cross section of groups for the elderly. They are conducted in many different settings and are designed to counsel, rehabilitate, and resocialize, to reconstruct the psyche, or merely to comfort and maintain the individual at the highest level of functioning possible. Reflective of the heterogeneity of the aging population itself, the chapters in this monograph aptly illustrate the wide range of interests and needs of this rapidly growing segment of our society.

In chapter 1 Tross and Blum present a review of the literature to bring us up to date with what is happening in the field. They classify the groups into two major categories: insight therapy, subdivided into psychoanalytic, self psychology, and life review groups; and supportive therapy, subdivided into verbal/social rehabilitative groups and activity therapy aimed at reducing the stresses of aging, maintaining coping skills, bolstering self-esteem, and correcting distortions in the patients' views of the world. Tross and Blum make the point that while groups for the elderly are often designed for patients with similar problems, each person must be viewed and treated as unique. They emphasize that group therapy for the elderly, as for any other age group, should be culture specific and, where possible, should be conducted in the membership's primary language.

In organizing this monograph, we have made use of Tross and Blum's categories. The authors in Part II report on insight therapy groups. In Parts III and IV verbal/social and rehabilitative groups are described, Part III dealing with groups for ambulatory patients, Part IV with groups for institutionalized patients and their relatives. Part V describes the use of the arts in group therapy for the elderly. The monograph concludes with a description of a training program for mental health associates that provides experience in many of these methods and enlists the assistance of the elderly.

Benitez-Bloch starts off the second section by describing the treatment, in regular adult therapy groups, of active elderly patients living in the community. She stresses the beneficial intergenerational transferences that can occur when patients of different ages are treated together.

Lakin next outlines the different ways in which members function in groups composed entirely of the elderly or entirely of young adults. He and his students found that elderly group members tend to differentiate the elderly as a subgroup, demand more leader guidance, and disclose more intimate details about mutually expected problems, such as loneliness, rejection, and the fear of abandonment. Younger group members, by contrast, feel their problems are more unique, become more anxious, and hesitate to reveal themselves. They are more likely to express boredom in the group. The elderly, it was determined, are less interested in here-and-now group issues. In the light of these findings, Lakin recommends strategies to be adopted in leading groups for the elderly.

In chapter 4 Weiner and White describe their adaptation of Kohut's self psychology to the treatment of elderly persons living in the community. Unlike Bloch, they do not mix the generations. They stress the capacity of the therapist and the group to help patients improve their self-esteem and increase their individuation through mirroring, idealized parental transference onto the therapist and "twinship" with other group members.

Lothstein, also working within a Kohutian framework, details the progress, in a psychodynamic therapy group, of active elderly patients suffering from borderline and neurotic problems. He focuses particularly on the problems created by the patients' increased dependency and the resultant role reversal with their children. He also examines the struggle for separation–individuation after the loss of a spouse.

In the final chapter of Part II, Schloss uses classic psychodramatic techniques in working with the elderly. Frequently the group deals with stereotypes about aging. He describes the reactions of a seventy-one-year-old woman and other group members to her desire to go to college. Members share in each other's psychodramas. They become protagonists in their own failures. They may deal with age-specific issues such as dilemmas around retiring, or they may work through lifelong problems and deal with unfinished business.

Part III reports on supportive and rehabilitative groups and cognitive behavioral groups for individuals living in the community. In chapter 7 Matorin and Zoubok describe the establishment of a group for chronic patients who have been seen individually once a month for long-term maintenance. During the first year the group met once a month. Refreshments were served and the focus was on the reduction of isolation and the improvement of coping skills. During the second year the group met twice a month and became more psychotherapeutic. Members examined their feelings about disability and death. They discussed how to manage sexuality in old age and revealed their anxieties about strokes and heart attacks. Some members revealed that they rejected eyeglasses, hearing aids, and dentures as symbols of old age. There was increased focus on how to function and how to respond to stresses within the limitations imposed by aging.

In chapter 8 Fisher describes a group combining activities and discussion in order to reduce the loneliness and frustrations of elderly people living impoverished lives in a large city. He finds that the combination of verbal and nonverbal expressions of the problems experienced by the members assists in their resolution. Activities, such as arts and crafts and food preparation, stimulate the expression of feelings in group members who are otherwise reticent. At times activities and discussions are arranged to occur together, while at other times they are organized sequentially; Fisher has not, however, determined the advantage of one organization over the other. In addition, he encourages networking and mutual support outside the group. Unfortunately, he has found that because of the activities and the settings (one group was held in a nutrition center) funding has been difficult to maintain. Grants have terminated, and Medicaid reimbursement has required a medical orientation.

Hainer next describes groups for widows who must work through their grief and learn to live independently. Once the grief work is accomplished, members must reintegrate their selves and remake their lives. The group is problem-oriented and experiential and encourages self-help and mutual assistance.

Rathbone-McCuan uses group therapy in the treatment of elderly alcoholics. The groups are led by multidisciplinary teams using a cognitive behavioral approach. Probably about 10 percent of the elderly suffer from alcoholism. Some of these people have always been alcoholics and are survivors, often with multiple disabilities. However, other elderly persons become alcoholic late in life, either because of an increased sensitivity to alcohol or because they use the substance to blunt the pain of other problems. For these people group therapy has been found very useful. Whether the groups should be focused on the drinking problem or on the life situation is a matter of judgment. Rathbone-McCuan holds that the treatment of alcoholics should emphasize conscious material and should focus on key cognitive and behavioral problems. She includes family members in some of these groups.

The groups reported in Part IV are held in a variety of institutional settings. Goodman describes open-ended groups in an acute care hospital. A pilot group was developed in a small unit composed of twelve elderly patients, some of whom were very regressed and confused. Most were coping with depression and had been treated with ECT. The therapy focused on the strengths of the elderly and helped them improve their communication. Themes in the group reflected the loneliness and isolation of the elderly, their strong need for affiliation, their dependence and fear of dementia, and their guilt over being mentally ill. Therapists were cross-generational, the senior therapist serving as a role model for the patients.

At first the therapists experienced resistance from other staff, and members were often prevented from attending the group. Later, however, this decreased and it became possible to develop a second group. Relations between the institutional management and staff and the group therapists are mentioned as important factors in success or failure by all writers describing groups in institutions. Competition for the time, attention, and affection of the group members, as well as for prestige, is often expressed through the nonprovision of adequate space and time and through the erection of obstacles to attendance at group. Wiener, working in the Veterans Administration medical programs, writes about an open-ended group for terminally ill cardiac patients, all but one of whom are male. He too deals with institutional issues, examining the problems created by the lack of status of an open-ended group led by a nonmedical staff member in a medically dominated hospital. He describes the problems that group members, leaders, and staff experience in confronting the seriousness of the patients' illness.

Open-ended groups are very common in acute care and general hospitals, and the point needs to be made that these groups for limited-stay patients sharing a common set of problems develop a life of their own. Once a group culture has been established and accepted, issues are dealt with repetitively, over a series of sessions, so that most patients will encounter them at one meeting or another.

In chapter 13 Bienenfeld describes supportive groups for patients in a state hospital. In these groups two major themes recur: the fear of illness and death, and the losses patients have experienced and an attendant nostalgia for better times. These patients also struggle with the loss of independence; the group helps them to face up to staff who sometimes attempt to exert undue control. Therapists in hospitals often have roles and relationships with patients outside the group, and Bienenfeld insists that the group therapist help patients be clear about these different roles.

Chapters 14 and 15 examine the selection and treatment of demented patients and their care givers. Aronson provides a description of the psychological stress that relatives experience as loved ones stricken with irreversible dementia deteriorate before their eyes and discusses various factors that need to be taken into consideration in selecting relatives for supportive group therapy. She stresses that the diagnosis must be firmly established and that the patient's situation—at home or in an institution—will make a difference as to how useful a group for relatives will be. Relatives of institutionalized patients face problems very different from those encountered by family members caring for their loved ones at home.

Sidney Saul describes group therapy for confused and demented patients and for their relatives both in outpatient settings and in institutions. The aims of these groups are to reduce the confusion and depression from which many patients suffer and to assist them to cope optimally. He describes a group that started with patients in an inner circle and with relatives observing from an outer circle. After some time the relatives expressed interest in more active participation and joined the inner circle.

Part V describes the use of the arts in group psychotherapy with the elderly. Shura Saul leads off this section by describing the values of group therapy using the various arts. While words may be too heavy a burden for some elderly patients, she notes, creative expression projects the felt life and can relieve pent-up emotions. Creativity taps unused resources, improves the members' inner balance, and promotes a sense of fulfillment. In a second chapter she describes how she uses poetry to stimulate elderly patients. Sometimes her groups read poetry together, sometimes the members all contribute to the creation of a poem as the culmination of the group's common feelings, and sometimes members will bring in poems that express significant aspects of their lives.

In chapter 18 Samberg writes about dance therapy with the elderly. She emphasizes the increased sense of physical and psychological well-being engendered by movement. Frustrations and tensions are reduced and emotional expressiveness increased by dancing. Patients get in touch with themselves and their feelings and are more conscious of their body and its boundaries. Dancing with others supplies a sense of intimacy and togetherness. Activity is geared to the needs and capacities of each group member, and even the very disabled can participate.

In the next chapter Morrin presents a theoretical description, illustrated with case material, of art therapy groups for elderly mentally disturbed patients. She draws on many theoretical approaches —humanistic, gestalt, behavioral—to open up new horizons for group members, to foster a sense of mastery, and to increase their self-esteem. At times group members will create their own art, while at others they will engage in group productions that illustrate their relationships to each other and to common group themes.

Stern, in chapter 20, shows the development of drama techniques, formal and improvisional, in both institutional and outpatient settings. Like Fischer in chapter 8, she raises the issue of how activity therapies can be paid for when most reimbursement is medically based. We can empathize with their frustration when useful programs must be terminated for lack of funds; they question whether financial requirements should be permitted to destroy the delivery of needed treatment or to distort its staffing.

Part VI ends the monograph with Moerman's description of a community college training program for mental health associates preparing for work with the elderly. This program embodies many of the themes and approaches described more fully in other chapters. The training group helps students explore their attitudes to elderly people and to their own aging, as well as allowing them an understanding of group process and how it feels to be a group member. Verbal group interactions and activities are combined both in the treatment of active elderly people drawn from the community around the college and in the students' work with frail elderly in nursing homes and hospitals.

Widely ranging theoretical approaches are brought to bear on the group treatment of mental health problems in the elderly. However, most of the authors here agree that treatment should be carried on within a positive transference. Although many therapists have emphasized the importance of providing support in the group therapy of the elderly, several chapters in this volume report the achievement of considerable change not only in behavior and mood but, more fundamentally, in the ways individuals perceive themselves and relate to others. Sometimes lifelong conflicts have been resolved as patients face the transitions and adjustments required to live as an elderly person in American society.

A major difference between the elderly and the young is that the former have a long history behind them and the expectation of a shorter time to live. They are also likely to experience reduced rather than expanded capabilities. Western civilization is less likely to offer the elderly new opportunities for achievement. Tasks are most frequently to adjust to the present and create the most favorable conditions for the future. The young have most of their lives still in front of them, or so they hope. Consequently, young adults are more likely to spend time fantasying and planning for the future, whereas the elderly may gain satisfaction from reminiscing about the past and sharing common values and experiences with others of their own generation. Reminiscence therapy coupled with activities, tempered to the capacities of the group members, is very useful for the handicapped, depressed, or otherwise isolated individual.

The age of the therapist is overtly or implicitly an issue in these chapters. Most therapists are in their middle years. They tend to reinforce the generational role reversal in the minds of patients, although the extent to which therapists foster dependency will vary with the nature of the group. Lothstein describes how the patients in his groups tended particularly to denigrate the young female therapists and to call them "girls." Lakin, in comparing groups of older and younger adults, ran the older group as their contemporary while younger therapists ran the young adult groups. Linden and his cotherapist, by contrast, felt that the fact that they were younger and full of vitality was useful to their elderly hospitalized patients. They speculated that the arrangement enabled the patients to identify with their idealized selves. Both Linden and Shura Saul comment that older people do not see themselves as changed or as essentially different from the way they were when young. Sometimes the lack of congruence between inner feelings and the outer physical shell can be painful and disconcerting. Older people must learn to recognize how they are perceived by others and to deal with the stereotypes that society would impose on them.

The training of older and younger group therapists should include an understanding of their attitudes to aging and death, both their own and others', and must be adjusted to the age and experience of the trainees. Older therapists are much more immediately attuned to the problems of active elderly patients who are their contemporaries, and are less likely to evoke role reversal transferences. In groups made up of relatives of the very old and disturbed, they may encounter the same problems and frustrations they experienced with their own aged parents. Whatever the situation, therapists need to guard against countertransferences resulting from their own unresolved conflicts related to aging. Linden emphasizes the importance of recognizing one's own stereotypes about aging; these must be overcome if therapists are to help their elderly patients. Stimulating the interest of young and middle-aged therapists to conduct group therapy for the elderly is still a challenge, and we hope this book will go some way in overcoming the hesitations of those not already working with this population. For those readers who are already experienced, we hope we have presented some stimulating ideas which they may add to their treatment repertoire.

Part I
Review of the Literature

1

A Review of Group Therapy with the Older Adult: Practice and Research

SUSAN TROSS, Ph.D. and
JUNE E. BLUM, Ph.D.

A compelling rationale exists for the use of group therapy with the older patient. The frequent biopsychosocial nature of late-life presenting problems and syndromes may be viewed as a specific indication for group therapy. Group therapy is likely to be the treatment of choice for the problems of social isolation, feelings of inadequacy, and sense of anonymity arising from older adults' low status in a youth-oriented society. The group setting is a direct opportunity for camaraderie, social exercise, and meaningful interpersonal interaction often unavailable to the older person. The group may also provide a forum for personal feedback about individual problems—from which both consensus and cognitive alternatives may be obtained. In addition, depending on the patient's ego strength and motivation, group can provide an opportunity to work through unresolved conflicts to freer intra- and interpersonal feelings. Inherent in the above are Yalom's curative factors which are not age-bound (1975). In light of this, there has been a surge of clinical interest in applying group techniques not only to age-specific issues but to the ongoing characterological stresses of older adults, as well as to the problems of the frail elderly.

Recent reviews of the literature testify to the growing commitment of group therapists to meeting the problems of the diverse older population (Berkman, 1978; Burnside, 1978; Blum and Tross, 1980; Hartford, 1980; Gallagher, 1981; Parham, Priddy, McGovern, and Richman, 1982; Saul, 1983; Yesavage and Karasu, 1983; Killiffer,

3

Bennett, and Gruen, 1984; Myers, 1984; White and Weiner, 1986). In the following review the major group approaches to older adults will be presented, and the sparse empirical literature on their efficacy summarized.

Like individual psychotherapeutic approaches to the older adult, the group approaches fall principally into two categories: (1) insight-oriented therapy, and (2) supportive therapy. The approaches reflect differential psychologies of late adulthood. The insight-oriented approach is directed at the working through of lifelong emotional conflicts; the supportive approach defines the reparation of late-life stresses as its central task. More recently a third group approach, distinct from but related to supportive therapy, has been developed—cognitive-behavioral group therapy (Beck and Rush, 1978; Beck, Rush, and Shaw, 1979)—and a fourth theoretical approach, attribution theory (Jones and Davis, 1965), adopted from social psychology, is being given consideration for group intervention with the troubled elderly (Sparacino, 1978; Lakin, Oppenheimer, and Bremer, 1982; and Parham et al., 1982).

In part the insight/supportive distinction reflects a differential focus on, respectively, inpatient and outpatient populations. The approaches more nearly follow Kahana's three broad categories of older patients (1979), i.e., the *aging,* who represent a broad range of personality types affected by losses, the *intermediate* group, who are in crisis, and the *debilitated* aged. The treatment lines and categories are not as rigid as presented, for there are many treatment variations to meet the needs of this very heterogeneous population. The groupings are made for descriptive purposes only.

INSIGHT-ORIENTED GROUP THERAPY

There are two major forms of insight-oriented group therapy with the older patient: (1) analytic group therapy; (2) life review therapy.

Analytic Group Therapy

The application of psychoanalytic theory and methods to groups of older patients was pioneered by Linden (1953, 1954, 1955, 1957). His work provided some seminal conceptualizations of the later years of the life cycle (Linden and Courtney, 1953). Initially, to restore social and practical functioning, he applied psychoanalytic methods to inpatient groups of "chronically senile women" (Linden, 1953). The response to free association, mutual interpretations, and free expression was encouraging. However, in the initial phase of the group he found structured methods (including didactic lectures, turn-taking, calling on patients, probing, and successive ten-minute patient presentations) to be more stimulating. He continued to use the transference dynamic of the therapist as an omnipotent parent, commonly shared by these patients, as a foundation for building group cohesion. When he introduced the use of male and female cotherapists as (1) parental transference stimuli, (2) sex role models, and (3) models for opposite-sex object choice, conventional psychotherapy emerged. Linden's work thus introduced directive techniques into analytic practice, an innovation necessitated by the functional capacity of patients. Grotjahn (1955, 1978) viewed psychoanalytic group therapy as the preferred treatment for the older patient due to the potential for transference interpretation. He postulated that the older patient's constricted social life lent emotional primacy to their transference reactions. Hence for them "working through" was more aptly described as "living through." At the same time, he observed that the intense transference reactions of standard psychoanalysis were mitigated in the group setting, where they are diffused. He saw the potential for three types of transference: (1) to the therapist, (2) to the group as a unit, and (3) to individual peers. He emphasized sexuality as one core issue that emerged in unstructured discussions. Here the group therapist is charged with knowing how to correct two myths: "Old people do not live beyond 'sin' and they must not expect to function unchanged" (Grotjahn, 1978). The second issue to emerge is death. Two common functions of the wish to die were observed: (1) as hostility turned inward against the self, and (2) as a weapon for hostile provocation of family members. Pragmatically, he suggested that medical attention should be available for group members after the session. Thus, members can feel their complaints have been heard and group cohesion may be supported. Hence he underscored the group task as one of communication. He emphasized the utility of group therapy for nursing home populations, for whom the group could offer cognitive stimulation and emotional responsivity.

Krasner's work (1959, 1977) exemplifies the use of group therapy with the "young-old" (Neugarten, 1975). He pioneered analytically oriented group therapy with an older outpatient population at the Postgraduate Center. While he found the group modality to be successful with these patients, he turned, as did Jackson and Grotjahn (1958), to combined individual and group therapy as the treatment of choice. In individual therapy, Krasner (1977) reported, the older patient generally experiences the therapist as a child. The working through of this inverse transference reaction was viewed by Krasner as a gateway for the elder's therapeutic change. He recognized the multiplicity of therapeutic mechanisms accessible in the group setting. These included the mobilization of diverse individual transferences, family transference, and emotional mirroring among the group members. His adaptation of psychoanalytically oriented therapy included (1) forming a working alliance around present adaptational issues; (2) mobilizing transference reactions via free association; (3) analysis of resistance and acting out; and (4) interpretation and working through of early developmental conflicts. Krasner advocated age-segregated groups for elders due to variables shared in common. However, his stance was developmental rather than static. When appropriate, he had elders progressing from a homogeneous elderly group to a heterogeneous one. There they could use their newly won insights to work through intergenerational conflicts.

Berland and Poggi (1979) obtained evidence of the need for an analytic psychotherapy approach from the subjective judgment of group members. Ranging in age from seventy-two to ninety-nine, they were residents of a private retirement home who had been selected as appearing isolated or depressed. After a trial period of supportive group therapy, they altered their stance on the consensual advice of their patients. The therapists became less transparent and facilitated expression of feeling by using individual, group-as-a-whole, and transference interpretations. They noted the growth of insight and interpersonal relatedness with the therapy. Death and loss were salient themes. The therapists observed, contrary to ageist myths, that the older people in the group (1) wanted to change, (2) could use metaphor, (3) did not have faulty memories, and (4) were capable of forming deep attachments to others. Hence for these authors and others (Grotjahn, 1955; Meerloo, 1955; Linden, 1957; Blum and Tallmer, 1977; Krasner, 1977; King, 1980) countertransference, not chronological age per se, emerged as a limit on therapy for older adults.

The need for an integrated (i.e., both supportive and analytic) group approach to the older patient is emphasized by Levine and Poston (1980). Their subjects were female psychiatric outpatients sixty-five or older with severe characterological problems, especially depression, hypochondriasis, and narcissistic features. They were described as "chronic complainers" who used externalization and somatization as primary modes of conflict expression. After a thoughtful consideration of each patient's dynamics and negative individual therapy experience, the authors concluded that analytic group therapy, as postulated by Durkin-Glatzer (Kauff, 1979), would be a viable intervention for their patients. As Berland and Poggi observed, they found resistance to an intervention that differed from the needs of group members. In this instance the therapists were conceptually ahead of their narcissistic patients.

They terminated the formal group and introduced as an alternative an informal coffee lounge approach. This was created to provide direct gratification through refreshments, social contact, brief individual attention from the therapists, and a context for ventilation. In this atmosphere the members themselves spontaneously generated formal group discussion. The coffee lounge led to the group cohesion the leaders sought. On the basis of this development a weekly two-phase intervention emerged: (1) refreshment time in the coffee lounge; (2) formal group time in a separate area. As a result they resumed the more classical tasks of resistance and transference interpretation they had previously abandoned. Increasing capacities for insight and empathy with the treatment are reported. In effect, by adapting the unexpected importance of patients' early developmental needs, the group eventually made use of the analytic stance initially chosen.

Others promote the use of psychoanalytic methods in individual or group settings, according to individual need. They describe benefits from psychoanalytically oriented therapies in the areas of reality-testing, insight expressiveness, interpersonal relatedness, and the capacity for sublimation of psychosexual conflicts or narcissistic injuries of later adulthood. Baker (1985) viewed the aging as being stuck in earlier transitions (uncompleted developmental tasks). She applied dynamic group psychotherapy to an age cohort group of patients fifty-five and older. Her focus was Erikson's late-life task of ego integrity (1963) in conjunction with life review conceptualizations. She observed that the use of group transference and multiple individual transferences facilitated a range of changes from a reidentification of self to a decision to change maladaptive behavior.

Leszcz (Leszcz, Feigenbaum, Sadavoy, and Robinson, 1985; Sadavoy and Leszcz, 1987) described dynamic interactional group therapy with male nursing home residents ranging in age from seventy to ninety-five. Here group is presented as a valuable modality for isolated, depressed, and demoralized men. As there is a minimum of psychological sophistication among the group members, the therapist verbalizes what is difficult for the members to express and integrates their comments. Modifications in technique—i.e., the therapist is highly active and supportive with therapeutic transparency—are noted. Dynamically, Leszcz employs life review conceptualizations, current theories of narcissism (Kohut, 1971) and the role of narcissistic injuries (Kernberg, 1977; Modell, 1977; Lazarus, 1980), all in the service of enhancing an older person's efforts to maintain or restore self-esteem in a period of loss (Sorensen, 1986).

Life Review Group Therapy

Life span developmental psychology has helped redefine late adulthood as a period of heightened self-examination, retrospection, and existential resolution. Butler (1975) has postulated that decreasing practical demands and greater proximity to death press for dramatic personal growth in late adulthood. Thus older adults are thought to make the goals of identity consolidation, intimacy, and resolution of problematic issues more immediate during this period. His premise is that the older adult strives to attain these goals through the naturally occurring process of life review, which combines reminiscence, longitudinal perspective, and appreciation of the present. Based on the occurrence of this process, he considers the older adult not simply a *viable* but rather a *prime* candidate for life review psychotherapy. Life review psychotherapy consists of encouraging (1) reminiscence of one's life, (2) absolution from lingering past guilt, (3) articulation of positive personal values, and (4) resolution of intra- and interpersonal conflicts. Butler (1974, 1975) applied the life review method to both group and individual settings. He felt that group members might model, supplement and support the life review process.

Butler also discussed the relative benefits of age-segregated and integrated groups. In the age-segregated group, members are bound by common developmental tasks and frames of reference. In the age-integrated group they may directly confront and overcome the inequities of ageist bias among younger adults; they may eventually attain the esteem of experienced mentors (Butler and Lewis, 1977).

Lakin, Oppenheimer, and Bremer (1982) empirically observed the rationale for age homogeneous groups in the later years. In their study the variable of self-disclosure differentiated older subjects (ages sixty-five to eighty) from younger ones (ages eighteen to twenty-two). Identity security and the feeling that many of their problems are shared by peers are noted as facilitators of disclosure for the older members.

SUPPORTIVE GROUP THERAPY

Groups provide the setting for a wide variety of supportive therapies. These may be classified under two broad headings: (1) verbal/social therapies, and (2) rehabilitation/activity therapies.

Verbal/Social Group Therapies

One category of supportive group therapy for older adults may be characterized as social therapy. Within this category the therapy group is used chiefly as a compensatory resource against the often constricting social network of the older adult (Kalson, 1965). This is in keeping with Goldfarb's goal for groups of "aged" that concerns stimulation of personal activity, sociability, and social integration (1971).

Group process itself is offered as corrective and gratifying social experience. It may be used as a laboratory for the exercise of social skills that may have deteriorated from disuse or that may be newly required by such major stressors of late adulthood as bereavement, moves, and extended family disruption (Klein, LeShan, and Furman, 1965; Feil, 1967; Davis and Klopfer, 1977). The group may also function as a source of consensus and empathy around common phase-specific problems and methods of coping (Oberleder, 1966; Altholz, 1973; Petty, Moeller, and Campbell, 1976; Waters, Fink, and White, 1976). The focus of this therapy is present adaptation. Its goal is improvement in practical function, whether disrupted by acute crisis (Blank, 1974; Mayadas and Hink, 1974) or restricted by a chronic lifestyle factor such as institutionalization. In this context the goals of group therapy with older patients discussed by Yalom and Terrazas (1968) represent the concept of supportive therapy, i.e., focusing on strengths and realistic goal setting.

During the early 1950s several authors initiated supportive group therapy with older, chronically institutionalized patients. Silver (1950) described one of the earliest therapy groups for paranoid or senile psychotic female inpatients seventy to eighty years of age. After food and drink served to entice patients to therapy, group discussion was conducted around the salient current concerns of somatic symptoms, positive memories, economic complaints, loneliness, wishful fantasy, and rejection. Silver reported improvement in sociability, mood, and behavior management. Benaim (1957), like Silver, catalogued the emergence of key themes in older patient groups. These included symptoms, marital conflicts, nostalgia for childhood, and personal role. He observed a continuity among the thematic concerns of his older group and one ranging in age from seventeen to forty-five. Kastenbaum (1965) later supplemented group therapy sessions with wine and beer to encourage social contact and to reduce the need for medication in older inpatients. A positive effect was later demonstrated by outcome studies (Chien, Stotsky, and Cole, 1973; Chien, Tammi, and Schloss, 1973; Mishara and Kastenbaum, 1974). Finkel and Fillmore (1971) treated psychiatric inpatients in twice-weekly supportive group therapy. They conceptualized the group as a resource for social contact, consensus, information, and emotional expression and understanding. At the same time, it also served to increase reality orientation, task motivation, and social skills. The authors were able to clarify unresolved differential diagnoses, based on their behavioral observations in the group setting.

Adjustment to the common stressful life events of late adulthood has also long been the focus of supportive group therapy. As early as 1959, Ross emphasized the utility of the therapy group as a resource for supporting the often isolated older patient after the frequent acute crises of late adulthood. In effect, group methods have provided a major approach to the key stresses of later years. These include preretirement (Giordano and Giordano, 1984); retirement (Seguin, 1973; Mannian, 1974; Bolton, 1976); marital problems (Goldfarb, 1968, 1971; Richman, 1979); bereavement (Michaels, 1977; DeBor, Gallagher, and Lasker, 1983); alcoholism (Dunlop, Skorney, and Hamilton, 1982); cognitive impairment (Cook, 1984); relocation (Saul and Saul, 1974; Dye, 1982); resocialization (Barron, 1980; Saul, 1983); and sexuality (Kaas, 1981; Croft, 1982; Hermanova, 1983; Starr and Weiner, 1983; and stressors of the care givers (Altschuler, Jacobs, and Shiode, 1985; Schmidt and Keyes, 1985).

However, it is not within the scope of this paper to review problem-specific interventions; rather, examples of these methods are presented. Oberleder (1966) used a crisis intervention model to treat patients with newly diagnosed senile psychosis. They were seen once weekly during a six-month period. Psychotherapy was aimed at reducing exaggerated psychopathological reactions to organic deficits. Although Oberleder focused on current adjustment, she conceptualized the patient's symptoms as the characterological recapitulation of earlier conflicts, especially those of middle age. Discussion centered on the management of intolerable negative feelings, especially anger, fear, and guilt. Selective memory loss or confabulation of emotionally problematic stimuli were confronted as defensive distortions. Patients were helped to assume increasing control over reactive symptoms. Exercises, including mirror confrontation, verbal statements, or other techniques, were used to further "unblock" perceptual functions. As patients neared readiness for discharge, they were transferred to a "hotel" ward as preparation for reentry into the community. The therapist also acted as liaison both to housing and senior center administrators and to families of patients. At termination all patients were able to be discharged from hospital and placed in other residential situations. Saul and Saul (1974) used a crisis-oriented therapy group to help patients cope with recent home relocation. They led group discussions around daily life in the nursing home, aimed at increased sense of familiarity and ease of adjustment. The group met once weekly for an hour and a half. They regarded group therapy as the treatment of choice, as an analog to the group living feature of nursing home residence. They emphasized the importance of the therapist characteristics of activity and preparedness (vis-à-vis prior session material).

Williams, Roback, and Pro (1980) described the process and outcome of a supportive problem-solving group for nonpsychiatric elderly women. The members were residents of a retired teachers' apartment complex who ranged in age from seventy-two to eighty-eight. Interpretations, particularly transference ones, were rare. A three-year follow-up investigation supported the impression that the group effort had been positive. Members were more aware of their feelings and had started to reestablish social and family ties. Williams and his colleagues felt Yalom's curative factors (1975) to be a contributing force. They concluded that the effectiveness of a group may be determined more by the therapists' attitude toward the aged than by their theoretical stance or professional background.

Some supportive therapists have proposed methods of group

therapy that reflect intermediary positions between supportive and insight-oriented extremes. Liederman, Green, and Liederman (1967) conducted unstructured group discussions from which they summarized the implications for realistic adaptation at the end of each session. They demonstrated that in combination with pharmacotherapy, outpatient groups could preclude otherwise imminent hospitalization. They also reported a reduction in paranoid and anxiety symptoms and an increase in extroversion.

Lesser, Lazarus, Frankel, and Havasu (1981) found that an eleven-week traditional psychotherapy program was unsuccessful with psychotic elderly patients. Improvement was obtained when they shifted to reminiscence group therapy. There group cohesion was obtained. Other authors, including Slavson (1964), rejected the use of reconstructive techniques with older adults. They viewed the older adult as a fragile dependent patient whose defenses required reinforcement rather than dismantling. Schwartz and Goodman (1952) conducted groups with elderly diabetics based on leader functions of instruction, judgment of progress, and authoritarian discipline (praise or criticism). Wolff (1963, 1970) emphasized the protective aspect of rigidity in the older patient. He used supportive group therapy for the resocialization of older adult inpatients. Within one year of treatment, 50 percent of his population was discharged from the hospital; over the next fifteen years they continued to demonstrate improvement on psychological tests and psychiatric examinations. Shere (1964) reemphasized the impact of social contact and empathic support in group work with older patients. She described activity, compassion, and flexibility as critical therapist qualities. She observed improvement in self-esteem, cognition, and interpersonal relations and a decrease in depressive symptoms in once-weekly group therapy.

Goldfarb (1971, 1974, 1975) was among the first to engage the elderly in couples group therapy. He observed the marital problems of aging couples to emerge from a search (successful or unsuccessful) by both or one partner for aid or support from the other. He consistently emphasized resources rather than deficits and stimulated social relationships and individual responsibility. This was exemplified in his manipulation of transference in the elderly. He used the omnipotent authority role his patients generally attributed to him to protectively set the stage for the patients to release their hopelessness and grievances. Thus, the patient was slowly guided to "transfer" his sense of power in the leader into a sense of his own personal effectiveness and to maintain the therapist as an ally. Goldfarb and Turner (1953) use this stance in brief therapy with inpatients suffering chronic brain damage. For others they recommend interventions applicable to the treatment of psychoneuroses and psychoses regardless of age.

Goldfarb, Linden, and others were of the opinion that transferences of the elderly differed from those of the young. Van der Kolk (1983) observed that the intensely idealized transference reactions arise during childhood and old age. In the elderly they are directed to the primary caregiver as a defense against feeling isolated. Hence van der Kolk, like Grotjahn, views group psychotherapy with "psychiatrically impaired elderly patients" as an opportunity to dilute the transference. With the reestablishment of peer relationships, dependency is mitigated and autonomy enhanced. Blau and Berezin (1982) contend that early object ties and level of maturity determine the type of transference more than does chronological age. The transferences of the earlier years are not so much different as broadened in scope due to greater life experience (Meerloo, 1955).

Rehabilitation/Activity Therapies

A broad range of therapy groups have been included as part of the milieu therapy offered by comprehensive geriatric treatment programs. Much of this therapy was initiated in inpatient settings with the goal of improving basic self-help skills or effecting hospital discharge. Rechtschaffen, Atkinson, and Freeman (1954) ran an inpatient therapeutic community for older patients combining supportive group and individual therapy, occupational therapy, recreational therapy, and ward work. They obtained a discharge rate three times greater than the pretreatment rate. However, at follow-up retesting no improvement was demonstrated on behavior rating scales. Pretreatment patient behavior and family involvement were found to be predictors of treatment outcome. Honigfeld, Rosenblum, Blumenthal, Lambert, and Roberts (1965) treated schizophrenic inpatients with medication and socialization group therapy. They obtained improvement in cooperativeness, grooming, motor function, and irritability. McNeil and Verwoerdt (1972) conducted therapy groups as part of a work program using inpatients fifteen to sixty-seven years of age as counselors on a geriatric unit. Kahana (1975) conducted problem-solving groups with both ambulatory health care facility residents and community center members. Groups met for five one-hour sessions. Using first hypothetical and then actual problems, the group focused on imparting basic problem-solving skills. These included information seeking, requests for assistance, and the use of external resources. He contrasted the interpersonal orientation of the community group with the concern with basic needs of the institutionalized group. Toseland (1977) also conducted problem-solving workshops with older adults, for whom he reported improvement in effective behavior. Sandel (1978) treated severely depressed, disoriented, wheelchair-bound chronic residents of a convalescent home in movement therapy groups. The patients ranged in age from seventy-seven to ninety-one. Techniques included rhythmic tasks with music, discussion and reminiscence, touch exercises for symbolic giving, and aggressive movement tasks. Whereas earlier they had typically been oppositional, withdrawn, and dissatisfied, they now made substantial gains in sociability, assertiveness, and spontaneous communication.

Koch (1977) viewed the tendency for reminiscence as a creative asset of this population. He conducted poetry workshops with nursing home residents. At each session he presented a key idea upon which the group members would improvise aloud. Koch would record their ordinary speech in poetry form. He observed an improvement in mood as a result of the emotional expression afforded them by poetry writing.

Saul's edited volume (1983) is addressed to creative group approaches in working with the frail elderly. Supportive, experiential, and educational group experiences are described, and goals are determined by specific types of frailty. There is a chapter that attends to relocation trauma and two papers pertaining to groups for caretakers (relatives and friends). Lowy, in his chapter, expresses the collection's theme and that of this review. Group experiences provide a "microcosm of the world" in which older adults have the opportunity to resolve conflicts related to individual needs.

In recent years increasing emphasis has been placed on the development of mental health programs for older patients. While not young in age, this population is, contrary to myths and stereotypes, responsible, verbal, intelligent, and sensitive, and describe wanting more for themselves. This group is not only getting older, it is also getting younger!

Turbow (1969) combined group therapy, structured activities, and day care in the treatment of outpatients sixty-one to eighty-nine who presented with emotional and physical complaints. These patients achieved a decrease in anxiety and an improvement in social interaction. Group members continued to maintain their own households during the three-year study. Granick (1975) reported decrements in anxiety, fears, and sense of inadequacy in older patients treated in combined discussion and activity groups. He also recommended psychodrama, encounter, and T-group methods as potentially effective means of therapeutic change in older adults' relationship skills. Berger and Berger (1973) founded the Center for Adults Plus as a day hospital for ambulatory patients with cognitive impairment. They offered a comprehensive regimen based on patient assessment and comprised of insight-oriented, socialization, and cognitive rehabilitation groups. Groups met three times weekly for three hours. During the first hour the authors conducted psychoanalytically oriented group psychotherapy; for the next two hours they used musical techniques, body movement tasks, and free association work exercises. Barnes, Sack, and Shore (1973) included group psychotherapy, psychodrama, world events discussion, resocialization (based on cooperative games like Scrabble, dominoes, or bridge), field trips, physical rehabilitation, and eating, cooking, and nutritional instruction. They reported increased social facility, sense of individual responsibility, and practical skill functioning as a result of treatment. Lieberman and Gourash (1979) have reported their effects of combining multidisciplinary humanistic techniques within a group for older people—SAGE (Senior Actualization and Growth Exploration). The changes achieved were not statistically significant. However, myths of aging were dispelled for participants and mental health scores improved.

Cognitive-Behavioral Group Therapy

Recent attention has been given to the application of cognitive-behavioral techniques to the group treatment of the older patient (Gallagher, 1981; Steuer and Hammen, 1983; Steinmetz, Thompson, Breckenridge, and Gallagher, 1985). To a large extent this is due to the fact that this modality was originally developed for the treatment of depression (Beck and Rush, 1978). As depression is a chief psychiatric complaint of older patients, this therapy may be considered particularly adaptable to this population. It also has the advantages of being time-limited, structured, and practical. In the group setting patients may function as adjunct therapists, identifying problem cognitions and behaviors and developing corrective strategies for them. Cognitive-behavioral therapy postulates that distortions in thinking underlie psychological symptoms. The immediate goal of therapy is the patient's recognition and correction of these distortions. This goal may be accomplished by a variety of cognitive techniques, such as graded task assignments, cognitive rehearsal, assertiveness training role-playing, and mood graphs (Gallagher and Thompson, 1982). The long-term goal of therapy is the modification of the implicit schemata or lifelong perspectives that make particular individuals prone to negative distortions. This goal may require repeated successes in correcting these distortions before the schemata are altered. Studies with older patients have reported significant decrements in depressive symptoms during cognitive-behavioral group therapy, results comparable to those obtained with more established treatments. Since these studies fall under the category of empirical outcome research, they will be reviewed with other studies of this type in a section to follow.

Sparacino (1978) has explored additional methods of facilitating cognitive change in elderly persons undergoing individual therapy. He borrowed attributional theory from social psychology (Jones and Davis, 1965) as a basis for intervention with the isolated. The therapeutic goal is to change an elderly person's negative debilitating self- and/or external attributions, which often become fixed as a result of diminished access to social consensus. Group, by affording opportunities for "sharing and comparing," is a natural medium for examining and changing attributions (Lakin, Oppenheimer, and Bremer, 1982; Parham et al., 1982).

ETHNIC VARIABLES IN GROUP THERAPY

A special issue in the group therapy interventions reviewed here are cultural and ethnic factors. Until recently, there have been few studies in this area. Kiev (1972) addressed these factors generally. Manuel (1982) discusses the sociological and social psychological issues in minority aging. Sue (1981) and Ridly (1984) focus respectively on counseling the culturally different and on clinical treatment of the nondisclosing black client. Ruiz (1975b) chaired a symposium on group therapy with minority group patients. He described the corrective impact of supportive group therapy on characterological problems. Age was not explicitly mentioned, and the considerations were not age-segregated. Elsewhere he addressed the influence of bilingualism on communication in groups (Ruiz, 1975a). He stressed the importance of using the patient's native tongue. This is invaluable for the older patient, whose basic values are imprinted in the primary language.

Dibner (1982) has discussed ethnic and cultural variations in the care of the aged. Lightfoot (1982) has succinctly presented the double jeopardy position of the black elderly, who are burdened not only by myths and stereotypes regarding the elderly, but also with negative racist stereotypes. Dunkas and Nikelly (1975) have focused on the adaptation of immigrants from diverse cultures to new cultural environments—with special attention to Greek immigrants. Szapacznik, Kurtines, Santisteban, and Perez-Vidal (1982) have proposed a "life enhancement counseling" technique for individual therapy with elderly patients which is adaptable to groups. They extended life review therapy to include an ecological component consisting of assessment and planned change of the transactions between the person and the environment.

Werbin and Hynes (1979) followed a group of Latino women patients between the ages of twenty and seventy for two years. They concluded that minority groups do not require different therapeutic approaches. A recent study by Franklin and Kaufman (1982) documented the applicability of group therapy with elderly Hispanic female patients. The group leader was a Venezuelan social worker familiar with Hispanic culture. As with Levine and Poston (1980), discussions shifted from emotional and physical complaints to more insightful issues. Falecov and Kaner (1984) stress the need for therapists to be culturally attuned. They present cultural strategy interventions which they used with Mexican-American families, including cultural reframing, cultural rituals, cultural family arrangements, language usage, cultural philosophy, and cultural remedies. Knowledge of values, customs, and ways of interacting of group members from diverse cultures and ethnic backgrounds is the sine qua non of group therapy.

GROUP THERAPY OUTCOME STUDIES

Despite the relative lack of empirical (as opposed to anecdotal) literature on group therapy with the older patient, group is nonetheless the major modality for which gerontological outcome research exists. The simultaneous application of uniform techniques in the group setting permits the accrual of larger samples and the standardization of intervention methods that are prerequisite for empirical evaluation. The finding of improvement spans a variety of group techniques and a variety of subpopulations of older adults.

Beginning with early outcome measurement in the 1950s, rate of institutional discharge, clinician ratings of prosocial or antisocial behavior, and patient-scored mood scales have served as criteria for improvement. Kubie and Landau (1953) obtained increases in social involvement and intellectual functioning among elderly Old Age Assistance clients at a day recreation center. Rechtschaffen, Atkinson, and Freeman (1954), as noted, observed a tripling of discharge rates following group and milieu treatment of geriatric inpatients. Wolk and Goldfarb (1967) obtained increases in sociability in this type of patient after one year of group treatment. Their degree of improvement, however, was less than that of a schizophrenic comparison group. Under both diagnostic categories, long-stay and recently admitted patients improved. Gunn (1968) observed a rise in the number of leaves granted and a decline in incidents of nurse-rated disruption in an elderly psychiatric population as a result of ward meetings. At the same time he reported an increase in depressive symptoms that he attributed to the broadening of a sense of reality accompanying failure in defensive denial. Schwartz and Papas (1968) found that disease-specific group therapy aided coping with the symptoms of illness and concomitant anxiety in geriatric cardiovascular, stroke, or diabetes patients.

Zimberg (1969) obtained symptom relief, decrease in prescription of medication, improved physical health, and practical adjustment with group treatment of elderly inner city outpatients by paraprofessionals in a hospital psychiatry department. Burnside (1971) reported the effectiveness of two years of group treatment in reactivating communication and socialization in residents of a convalescent home. Manaster (1972) reported increased memory function, symptom relief, emotional expressiveness, sense of self, and adaptive behavior in elderly demented as a result of structured, supportive group therapy. Conrad (1974) reported a decline in social withdrawal in housing project residents following expressive group therapy. Paradis (1974) obtained symptom relief of sleeplessness and appetite loss in depressive patients following brief group therapy that was supportive and directive; at the same time their physical appearance and socialization improved.

A few studies have examined the comparative impact of specific group techniques on the older patient. Nevruz and Hrushka (1969) compared outcome in structured and nonstructured groups. When discharge rates were used as measures, there were no differences between the groups. However, they observed greater interpersonal bonds among the members of the unstructured group, as evidenced by a higher degree of recall of names.

Ingersoll and Silverman (1978) investigated the relative effectiveness of behavioral and insight-oriented therapy groups meeting once weekly for eight weeks. Their subjects were volunteer community-dwellers who presented with anxiety, depression, and memory problems. A "here-and-now" technique based on relaxation, memory, and self-awareness tasks was compared to a "there-and-then" life review technique using genograms, journals, and discussion. Both methods obtained increases in self-esteem. However, only the life review subjects showed improvement in anxiety and physical symptoms.

Steuer and her colleagues (Steuer, Mintz, and Jarvik, 1982; Steuer, Mintz, Hammen, Hill, Jarvik, McCarley, Motoike, and Rosen, 1984) compared the outcomes of cognitive-behavioral group therapy and psychodynamic group therapy. Their subjects were community volunteers who met the DSM-III criteria for Major Depressive Disorder and had minimum Cutting scores on observer-rated and self-report depression scales. Ten subjects per therapy condition attended at least twenty-six of forty-six hour-and-a-half therapy sessions conducted on a once- or twice-weekly basis over a nine-month period. Both groups demonstrated clinically and statistically significant decrements in observer-rated and self-reported depression and anxiety. The cognitive-behavioral group showed significantly greater improvement than the psychodynamic group on the single parameter of the Beck Depression Inventory. However, this difference was not clinically significant, and was interpreted as an artifact of the inventory's ideational content. Rather, the authors concluded that both therapy conditions were equally effective in producing meaningful symptom relief. They also emphasized the critical association between treatment compliance and efficacy in demonstrating that the incidence of remission was almost solely confined to the subgroup of patients who were "completers" (those who attended at least twenty-six sessions). Thus the group therapy outcome literature with older patients corroborates the finding of uniform benefit for all comparative treatment arms that characterizes the psychotherapy outcome literature in general (Luborsky, Singer, and Luborsky, 1976). This finding is probably best explained as a function of the "nonspecific" ingredients that these therapies share, including therapist attention, interpersonal contact, and empathy (Frank, 1976).

When drug regimens and group techniques are studied comparatively, group treatment yields less promising results. Williams, Csalany, and Misevic (1967) assigned sixty-four older psychiatric inpatients to four conditions, including drug only, drug plus group discussion, group only, and control. They obtained improvement only in the combined drug plus group discussion. Chien (1971) randomized forty geriatric inpatients, a majority of whom were diagnosed as cognitively impaired, into four treatment arms. They included (1) beer and social "pub," (2) nonalcoholic punch and social "pub," (3) thioridazine punch and social "pub," and (4) thioridazine only, administered in the routine ward setting. On measures of both symptom relief and sociability, the beer condition yielded the most improvement and the "pub" condition the least. Similarly, Carroll (1979) obtained consistent improvement on socialization and ward activity (including response to recreational, occupational, and music therapy) for drink plus social hour subjects versus erratic improvement for nondrinkers.

More recently Jarvik, Mintz, Steuer, and Gerner (1982) compared the effects of tricyclic antidepressants, placebo drug treatment, and group psychotherapy in older depressed outpatients. The antidepressant condition combined twelve patients receiving doxepin and ten receiving imipramine, as the two subgroups showed similar benefit from therapy. The group psychotherapy condition combined fourteen patients in cognitive-behavioral group and twelve in psychodynamic group, as these subgroups showed similar benefit from therapy. The outcome period was the first twenty-six weeks of therapy. Both antidepressant and group therapy resulted in greater symptomatic improvement than the placebo drug condition. However, this improvement was greater for the antidepressant condition than for the group therapy condition, when rates of complete remission or of mean magnitude of symptom scale decrements were analyzed.

The Jarvik, Mintz, Steuer, and Gerner study was an interim analysis. Steuer, Mintz, and Jarvik (in press) reported that end point results revealed contradictory results. For example, group therapy outcome appeared to be as effective as the antidepressants on the Beck Depression Inventory. This was not the case when Hamilton Depression Rating Scale (1960) and Zung Self-Rated Depression Scale (1965) scores were analyzed. The authors conjecture that the Beck scale items are concerned with cognition and feelings which respond to psychotherapy, while the Hamilton and Zung items, heavily weighted toward the somatic, respond best to drug treatment. Thus, the researchers concluded that if the two treatment interventions—psychotherapy and pharmacological therapy—are treating different aspects of depression, their combination could be the intervention of choice in older patients. This has been demonstrated for younger patients by DiMascio, Weissman, Prusoff, New, Zwilling, and Klerman (1979).

As is the case with practitioners of clinical gerontology, group leaders come from many disciplines, including medicine, psychiatry, psychology, social work, and nursing. In addition, there are self-help groups such as those for widows (Silverman, 1978) and groups led by paraprofessionals. Evaluation of the latter interventions is being conducted. Outcome studies comparing leadership effectiveness are now being reported. Gallagher (1981) compared the effectiveness of professionals and nonprofessionals as instructors for classes of depressed elderly persons. Their goal was to prevent depression or to ameliorate current distress through the implementation of behavior skills. Members improved in overall morale. However, leader competence was determined more by willingness and ability to apply the behavioral/psychoeducational approach consistently and accurately than by professional status per se. Lieberman and Blivise (1985) compared the effectiveness of peer-directed and professionally directed groups for the elderly. Like Thompson, Gallagher, Nies, and Epstein (1983), they reported both leadership interventions to be valuable. However, the peer-led groups were not as effective as the professionally led ones.

CONCLUSION

Group therapy has gained increasing importance in the treatment of psychological problems of later adulthood. Clinical efforts have encompassed a broad range of techniques, including insight, existential, and support orientations and verbal and sensorimotor modalities in both inpatient and outpatient settings. The results of evaluative studies replicate those of psychotherapy in general. That is, most forms of therapy appear to produce greater improvement in symptoms than no treatment or placebo treatment. However, no single form of treatment has proven more effective than any other. This lack of differentiation may in part be an artifact of the relative novelty of these therapies and their lack of specificity; further research is needed to detect the comparative efficacy of individual treatments for individual problems. Alternatively, these results may reflect the true finding of generalized amenability to group therapy in older adults. The older adult may stand to benefit particularly from group therapy, given age-specific ego assaults and narcissistic issues. It may be that the "nonspecific" opportunity for camaraderie and consensus afforded by any of the groups means that it is the most powerful agent of therapeutic change. The widespread positive effects demonstrated for the group therapies provide yet another body of evidence in support of psychological development in late adulthood that attends to social, cultural, and ethnic variables.

REFERENCES

Altschuler, J., Jacobs, S., & Shiode, D. (1985), Psychodynamic time-limited groups for adult children of aging parents. *Amer. J. Orthopsychiat.*, 55:397–404.

Altholz, J. (1973), Outpatient group therapy with the elderly person. *Gerontologist*, 13:101–106.

Baker, F. M. (1985), Group psychotherapy with patients over 55: An adult development approach. *J. Geriatric Psychiat.*, 17:79–84.

Barnes, E. K., Sack, A., & Shore, H. (1973), Guidelines to treatment approaches. *Gerontology*, 13:513–517.

Barron, E. (1980), Initial reactions of newcomers of a residential setting for the aged to a resocialization program: An exploratory study. In: *Aging, Isolation and Resocialization*, ed. R. Bennett. New York: Van Nostrand Rheinhold, pp. 152–168.

Beck, A. T., & Rush, A. J. (1978), Cognitive approaches to depression and suicide. In: *Cognitive Defects in the Development of Mental Illness*, ed. C. Serban. New York: Brunner/Mazel, pp. 235–258.

———— ———— Shaw, B. F. (1979), *Cognitive Therapy of Depression*. New York: Guilford.

Benaim, S. (1957), Group psychotherapy within a geriatric unit: An experiment. *Internat. J. Social Psychiat.*, 3:123–128.

Berezin, M. A. (1972), Psychodynamic considerations of aging and the aged: An overview. *Amer. J. Psychiat.*, 128:1483–1497.

Berger, L. F., & Berger, M. M. (1973), A holistic group approach to psychogeriatric outpatients. *Internat. J. Group Psychother.*, 23:432–444.

Berkman, B. (1978), Mental health and the aging: A review of the literature for clinical social workers. *Clin. Social Work J.* 6:230–245.

Berland, D. I., & Poggi, R. (1979), Expressive group psychotherapy with the aging. *Internat. J. Group Psychother.*, 29:87–108.

Blank, M. D. (1977), Meeting the needs of the aged: The social worker in the community health center. *Public Health Reports*, 92:39–42.

Blank, M. L. (1974), Raising the age barrier to psychotherapy. *Geriatrics*, 1:141–148.

Blau, D. and Berezin, M. A. (1982), Neuroses and character disorders. *J. Geriatric Psychiat.*, 15:55–95.

Blum, J. E., & Tallmer, M. (1977), The therapist vis-à-vis the older patient. *Psychotherapy: Theory, Research & Practice*, 14:361–367.

———— Tross, S. (1980), Psychodynamic treatment of the elderly: A review of issues in theory and practice. In: *Annual Review of Gerontology & Geriatrics*, ed. C. Eisdorfer. New York: Springer, pp. 204–237.

———— Weiner, M. B. (1979), Neuroses in the older adult. In: *Psychopathology of the Aging*, ed. O. J. Kaplan. New York: Academic Press, pp. 314–351.

Bolton, C. R. (1976), Humanistic instructional strategies and retirement education programming. *Gerontologist*, 16:550–555.

Burnside, I. M. (1971), Long-term group work with the hospitalized aged. *Gerontologist*, 11:213–218.

———— (1978), *Working with the Elderly: Group Processes and Techniques*. North Scituate, Mass.: Duxbury Press.

Butler, R. N. (1974), Successful aging and the role of the life review. *J. Amer. Geriatrics Soc.*, 22:529–535.

———— (1975), Psychiatry and the elderly: An overview. *Amer. J. Psychiat.*, 132:893–900.

———— Lewis, M. I. (1977), *Aging and Mental Health: Psychosocial Approaches*. St. Louis: Mosby.

Cacciola, E. J. (1982), Some aspects of working with the Italian elderly. *J. Geriatric Psychiat.*, 15:197–209.

Carroll, P. J. (1979), The social hour for geropsychiatric patients. *J. Amer. Geriatric Soc.*, 26:32–35.

Chien, C. P. (1971), Psychiatric treatment for geriatric patients: "Pub or Drug?" *Amer. J. Psychiat.*, 127:1070–1074.

———— Stotsky, B., & Cole, J. O. (1971), Psychiatric treatment for nursing home patients: Drug, alcohol and milieu. *Amer. J. Psychiat.*, 130:543.

———— Tammi, J., & Schloss, P. (1973), Beer and wine as incentives in a work therapy program. *Hospital & Community Psychiat.*, 130:99.

Cohen, P. M. (1983), A group approach for working with families of the elderly. *Gerontologist*, 23:248–250.

Conrad, W. K. (1974), A group therapy program with older adults in a high-risk neighborhood setting. *Internat. J. Group Psychother.*, 24:358–360.

Cook, J. B. (1984), Reminiscing: How it can help confused nursing home residents. *Social Casework*, 65(2):90–93.

Cosin, et al., (1958), Experimental treatment of persistent senile confusion. *Internat. J. Social Psychiat.*, 4:24.

Croft, L. H. (1982), *Sexuality in Later Life: A Counselling Guide for Physicians*. Boston: John Wright.

Davis, R. W., & Klopfer, W. G. (1977), Issues in psychotherapy with the aged. *Psychotherapy: Theory, Research & Practice*, 14:343–348.

DeBor, L., Gallagher, D., & Lasker, E. (1983), Group counseling with bereaving elderly. *Clin. Gerontologist*, 1(3):81–90.

Delgado, M. (1982), Hispanic elderly and natural support systems. *J. Geriatric Psychiat.*, 15:239–253.

———— (1983). Hispanics and psychotherapeutic groups. *Internat. J. Geriatric Psychother.*, 33:507–520.

Dibner, A. S. (1982). Ethnic and cultural variations in the care of the aged: Introduction. *J. Geriatric Psychiat.*, 15:193–196.

DiMascio, A., Weissman, M. M., Prusoff, B. A., New, C., Zwilling, M., &

Klerman, G. (1979), Differential symptom reduction by drugs and psychotherapy in acute depression. *Arch. Gen. Psychiat.*, 36:1450–1456.

Duffy, M. (1984), Aging and the family. *Psychother.*, 21:342–347.

Dunkas, N., & Nikelly, A. G. (1975), Group psychotherapy with Greek immigrants. *Internat. J. Group Psychother.*, 25:402–409.

Dunlop, J., Skorney, B., & Hamilton, J. (1982), Group treatment for elderly alcoholics and their families. *Social Work with Groups*, 5:87–92.

Dye, C. (1982). The experience of separation at the time of placement in long-term care facilities. *Psychother.*, 19:532–533.

Erikson, E. (1963), *Childhood and Society*, rev. ed. New York: Norton.

Evans, R. L., Werkhoven, W., and Fox, H. R. (1982), Treatment of social isolation and loneliness in a sample of visually impaired elderly persons. *Psychological Reports*, 5:103–108.

Falecov, C. J., and Kaner, B. M. (1984), Therapeutic strategies for Mexican-American families. *Internat. J. Fam. Ther.*, 6:18–30.

Feil, W. W. (1967), Group therapy in a home for the aged. *Gerontologist*, 7:192–195.

Finkel, S., & Fillmore, W. (1971), Experiences with an older adult group at a private psychiatric hospital. *J. Geriatric Psychiat.*, 4:188–199.

Frank, J. (1976), Psychotherapy and the sense of mastery. In: *Evaluation of Psychological Therapies*, ed. R. L. Spitzer & D. F. Klein. Baltimore: Johns Hopkins University Press.

Franklin, G. S., & Kaufman, K. S. (1982), Group psychotherapy for elderly female Hispanic outpatients. *Hospital & Community Psychiat.*, 33:385–387.

Gallagher, D. (1981), Behavioral group therapy with elderly depressives: An experimental study. In: *Behavioral Group Therapy*, ed. D. Upper & S. Ross. Champaign, IL: Research Press, pp. 187–224.

—————— Thompson, L. (1978), Conceptual and clinical issues in the psychotherapy of elderly depressed persons. Paper presented at the Annual Meeting of the Society for Psychotherapy Research, Toronto.

—————— —————— (1982), Treatment of major depressive disorders in older adult outpatients with brief psychotherapies. *Psychotherapy: Theory, Research & Practice*, 4:482–490.

Giordano, J. A., & Giordano, N. H. (1984). A classification of preretirement teams: In search of a new model. *Educational Gerontology*, 9(2–3):123–137.

Goldfarb, A. I. (1955), Psychotherapy of aged persons: One aspect of the psychodynamics of the therapeutic situation with aged patients. *Psychoanal. Rev.*, 42:180–187.

—————— (1968), Marital problems of older persons. In: *The Marriage Relationship*, ed. S. Rosenbaum & I. Alger. New York: Basic Books, pp. 105–119.

—————— (1971), Group therapy to the old and aged. In: *Comprehensive Group Therapy*, ed. H. I. Kaplan & B. J. Sadock. Baltimore: Williams & Wilkins, pp. 623–642.

—————— (1974), Minor maladjustments of the aged. In: *American Handbook of Psychiatry*, ed. S. Arieti & E. B. Brody. New York: Basic Books, 13:193–198.

—————— (1975), Integrated services. In: *Modern Perspectives in the Psychiatry of Old Age*, ed. J. G. Howells. New York: Brunner/Mazel, pp. 540–569.

—————— Turner, H. (1953), Psychotherapy of aged persons. *Amer. J. Psychiat.*, 109:906–915.

Granick, S. (1975), Group and family therapies with the aged. Paper presented at a symposium on Psychotherapy With the Aged: Annual Meeting of the American Psychological Association, Chicago.

Grotjahn, M. (1955), Analytical psychotherapy with the elderly. *Psychoanal. Rev.*, 42:419–427.

———— (1978), Group communication and group therapy with the aged: A promising project. In: *Aging into the Twenty-first Century: Middle-Agers Today*, ed. L. F. Jarvik. New York, Gardner Press, pp. 113–121.

Gunn, J. C. (1968), An objective evaluation of geriatric ward meetings. *J. Neurol., Neurosurg. & Psychiat.*, 31:403–407.

Hamilton, M. (1960), A rating scale for depression. *J. Neurol., Neurosurg. & Psychiat.*, 23:56–62.

Hartford, M. E. (1980), The use of group methods for work with the aged. In: *Handbook of Mental Health and Aging*, ed. J. E. Birrin & R. B. Sloane. Englewood Cliffs, N.J.: Prentice Hall.

Hermanova, H. M. (1983), Human sexuality and aging. In: *Aging in the Eighties and Beyond*, ed. M. Bergener, U. Lehr, E. Lang & R. Schmitz-Scherger. New York: Springer, pp. 324–333.

Honigfeld, G., Rosenblum, M., Blumenthal, I., Lambert, H., & Roberts, A. (1965), Behavioral improvement in the older schizophrenic patient: Drug and social therapies. *J. Amer. Geriatrics Soc.*, 13:57–72.

Ingersoll, B., & Silverman, A. (1978), Comparative group psychotherapy for the aged. *Gerontologist*, 18:201–206.

Jackson, J., & Grotjahn, M. (1958). The treatment of oral defenses by combined individual and group psychotherapy. *Internat. J. Group Psychother.*, 8:373–382.

Jarvik, L. F., Mintz, J., Steuer, J., & Gerner, R. (1982), Treating geriatric depression: A 26-week interim analysis. *J. Amer. Geriatrics Soc.*, 30:713–717.

Jones, E. E., & Davis, K. (1965). From art to disposition: The attribution process in person perception. In: *Advances in Experimental Social Psychology: Vol. 2*, ed. L. Berkowitz. New York: Academic Press, pp. 219–266.

Kaas, M. J. (1981), Geriatric sexuality breakdown syndrome. *Internat. J. Aging & Human Devel.*, 13:71–80.

Kahana, B. (1975), Training the aged for "competent coping": A psychotherapeutic strategy. Paper presented at the International Gerontological Meetings, Jerusalem.

Kahana, R. J. (1979), Strategies of dynamic psychotherapy with the wide range of older individuals. *J. Geriatric Psychiat.*, 12:71–101.

———— (1981), Reconciliation between the generations: A last chance. *J. Geriatric Psychiat.*, 14:225–239.

———— Krasner, J. D. (1977), Loss of dignity-courtesy of modern science. *Psychotherapy: Theory, Research & Practice*, 14:309–318.

Kalson, L. (1965), The therapy of discussion. *Geriatrics*, 20:397–401.

Kastenbaum, R. (1965), Wine and fellowship in aging: An exploratory action program. *J. Human Relations*, 13:266–275.

Kauff, P. F. (1979), Diversity in analytic group psychotherapy. *Internat. J. Group Psychother.*, 29:51–65.

Kernberg, O. (1977), The fate of narcissism in old age: Clinical case reports: Discussion. *J. Geriatric Psychiat.*, 10:27–45.

Kiev, A. (1972), *Transcultural Psychiatry*. New York: The Free Press.

Killiffer, E. H. P., Bennett, R., & Gruen, G. (1984), *Handbook of Innovative Programs for the Impaired Elderly*. New York: Haworth.

King, P. (1980), The life cycle as indicated by the nature of the transference in the psychoanalysis of the middle-aged and the elderly. *Internat. J. Psycho-Anal.*, 61:153–160.

Klein, W. H., LeShan, E. J., & Furman, S. S. (1965), *Promoting Mental Health of Older People Through Group Methods: A Practical Guide.* New York: Mental Health Materials Center.

Koch, L. (1977), *I Never Told Anybody: Teaching Poetry Writing in a Nursing Home.* New York: Random House.

Kohut, H. (1971), *The Analysis of the Self.* New York: International Universities Press.

Krasner, J. (1959), The psychoanalytic treatment of the elder person via group psychotherapy. *Acta Psychother.*, 7 (suppl):205–223.

————— (1977), Treatment of the elder person. In: *To Enjoy Is to Live,* ed. F. Fabricant, J. Barron, & J. Krasner. Chicago: Nelson Hall, pp. 191–204.

Kubie, S. H., & Landau, G. (1953), *Group Work with the Aged.* New York: International Universities Press.

Lakin, M., Oppenheimer, B., & Bremer, J. (1982), A note on old and young in helping groups. *Psychotherapy: Theory, Research & Practice,* 19:444–452.

Lazarus, L. W. (1980), Self psychology and psychotherapy with the elderly: Theory and practice. *J. Geriatric Psychiat.*, 13:69–88.

Lesser, J., Lazarus, L. W., Frankel, R. A., & Havasu, S. (1981), Reminiscence group therapy with psychotic geriatric inpatients. *Gerontologist,* 21:291–296.

Leszcz, M., Feigenbaum, E., Sadavoy, J., & Robinson, A. (1985), A men's group: Psychotherapy of elderly men. *Internat. J. Group Psychother.*, 35:177–196.

Levine, B. E., & Poston, M. (1980), A modified group treatment for elderly narcissistic patients. *Internat. J. Group Psychother.*, 30:153–167.

Lieberman, M. A., & Bliwise, M. D. (1985), Comparison of peer-professional directed groups for the elderly: Implications for the development of self-help groups. *Internat. J. Group Psychother.*, 35:155–175.

————— Gourash, N. (1979), Evaluating the effects of change groups on the elderly. *Internat. J. Group Psychother.*, 29:283–304.

Liederman, P. C., Green, R., and Liederman, V. R. (1967), Outpatient group therapy with geriatric patients. *Geriatrics,* 22:148–153.

Lightfoot, O. B. (1982), Psychiatric interventions with blacks: The elderly—a case in point. *J. Geriatric Psychiat.*, 15:209–225.

Linden, M. E. (1953), Group psychotherapy with institutionalized senile women: Study in gerontologic human relations. *Internat. J. Group Psychother.*, 3:150–170.

————— (1954), The significance of dual leadership in gerontologic group psychotherapy. *Internat. J. Group Psychother.*, 4:262–273.

————— (1955), Transference in gerontologic group psychotherapy: IV. Studies in gerontologic human relations. *Internat. J. Group Psychother.*, 5:61–79.

————— (1957), The promise of therapy in the emotional problems of aging. Paper presented at the Fourth Congress of the International Association of Gerontology, Merano, Italy.

————— (1963), The aging and the community. *Geriatrics,* 18:404–410.

————— Courtney, P. (1953), The human life cycle and its interruptions. *Amer. J. Psychiat.*, 109:906–915.

Luborsky, L., Singer, B., & Luborsky, L. (1976), Comparative studies of psychotherapy: Is it that "everybody has won and all must have prizes?" In: *Evaluation of Psychological Therapies,* ed. R. L. Spitzer & D. F. Klein. Baltimore: Johns Hopkins University Press, pp. 3–38.

Manaster, A. (1972), Therapy with the "senile" geriatric patient. *Internat. J. Group Psychother.*, 22:250–257.

Mannian, M. V. (1974), Issues and trends in preretirement education. *Industrial Gerontology*, 1:28–36.

Manuel, R. C. (1982), *Minority Aging: Sociological and Social Psychological Issues.* Westport, Conn.: Greenwood Press.

Mayadas, N., & Hink, D. (1974), Group work with the aged. *Gerontologist,* 14:440–445.

McNeil, J. N., & Verwoerdt, A. (1972), A group treatment program combined with a work project on the geriatric unit of a state hospital. *J. Amer. Geriatrics Soc.,* 20:259–264.

Meerloo, J. A. M. (1955), Transference and resistance in geriatric psychotherapy. *Psychoanal. Rev.,* 42:72–82.

Michaels, F. (1977), The effects of discussing grief, loss, death and dying on depressive levels in a geriatric outpatient therapy group. *Dissertation Abstracts Internat.,* 38(2–12):910.

Mishara, B. L., & Kastenbaum, R. (1974), Wine in the treatment of long-term geriatric patients in mental institutions. *J. Amer. Geriatrics Soc.,* 22:88–94.

Modell, A. M. (1977), The fate of narcissism in old age: Clinical case reports: Discussion. *J. Geriatric Psychiat.,* 10:47–53.

Myers, W. A. (1984), *Dynamic Therapy of the Older Patient.* New York: Aronson.

Neugarten, B. (1975), The future of the young-old. *Gerontologist,* 15:4–9.

Nevruz, N., & Hrushka, M. (1969), The influence of unstructured and structured group psychotherapy with geriatric patients on their decision to leave the hospital. *Internat. J. Group Psychother.,* 19:72–78.

Oberleder, M. (1966), Psychotherapy with the aging: An art of the possible? *Psychotherapy: Theory, Research & Practice,* 3:139–142.

——— (1970), Crisis therapy in mental breakdown of the aging. *Gerontologist,* 10:111–114.

Paradis, A. P. (1974), Brief outpatient group psychotherapy with older patients in the treatment of age-related problems. *Dissertation Abstracts Internat.,* 34(6–B):2947–2948.

Parham, I. A., Priddy, J. M., McGovern, T. V., & Richman, C. M. (1982), Group psychotherapy with the elderly: Problems and prospects. *Psychotherapy: Theory, Research & Practice,* 19:437–443.

Petty, B., Moeller, I., & Campbell, R. (1976). Support groups for elderly persons in the community. *Gerontologist,* 16:522–529.

Radebold, H. (1976), Psychoanalytic group psychotherapy with older adults: Report on specific issues. *Zeitschrift fur Gerontologie,* 9:128–142.

Rechtschaffen, A., Atkinson, S., & Freeman, J. G. (1954), Intensive treatment program for state hospital geriatric patients. *Geriatrics,* 9:28–34.

Richman, J. (1979), A couples theory group on a geriatric service. *J. Geriatric Psychiat.,* 12:203–213.

Ridly, C. R. (1984), Clinical treatment of the nondisclosing black client: A therapeutic paradox. *Amer. Psychologist,* 39:1234–1244.

Ross, M. (1959), Recent contributions to gerontologic group psychotherapy. *Internat. J. Group Psychother.,* 9:442–450.

Ruiz, E. J. (1975a), Influence of bilingualism on communication in groups. *Internat. J. Group Psychother.,* 25:391–395.

——— (1975b), Introduction to symposium: Group therapy with minority group patients. *Internat. J. Group Psychother.,* 25:389–390.

Sadavoy, J., & Leszcz, M. (1987), *Treating the Elderly with Psychotherapy: The*

Scope for Change in Later Life. Madison, Conn.: International Universities Press.

Sandel, S. L. (1978), Movement therapy with geriatric patients in a convalescent home. *Hospital & Community Psychiat.*, 29:738–741.

Saul, S., Ed. (1983), *Group Work with the Frail Elderly.* New York: Haworth.

Saul, S. R., & Saul, S. (1974), Group psychotherapy in a proprietary nursing home. *Gerontologist,* 14:446–450.

Schmidt, G. L., & Keyes, B. (1985), Group psychotherapy with family caregivers of demented patients. *Gerontologist,* 25:347–350.

Schwartz, E. D., & Goodman, J. I. (1952), Group therapy of obesity in elderly diabetics. *Geriatrics,* 7:280–283.

Schwartz, W., & Papas, A. T. (1968), Verbal communication in therapy. *Psychosomatics,* 9:71–74.

Seguin, M. M. (1973), Opportunity for peer socialization to old age in a retirement community. *Gerontologist,* 13:208–214.

Shere, E. (1964), Group therapy with the very old. In: *New Thoughts on Old Age,* ed. R. Kastenbaum. New York: Springer, pp. 146–160.

Silver, A. (1950), Group psychotherapy with senile psychotic patients. *Geriatrics,* 5:147–150.

Silverman, P. (1978), *Mutual Help Groups.* Washington, D.C.: NIMH.

Slavson, S. R. (1964), *A Textbook in Analytic Group Psychotherapy.* New York: International Universities Press.

Sorensen, M. H. (1986), Narcissism and loss in the elderly: Strategies for an inpatient older adults group. *Internat. J. Group Psychother.,* 36:533–549.

Sparacino, J. (1978), An attributional approach to psychotherapy with the aged. *J. Amer. Geriatrics Soc.,* 26:414–417.

Stabler, N. (1981), The use of groups in day centers for older adults. *Social Work with Groups,* 4(3–4):43–54.

Starr, B., & Weiner, M. B. (1983), The Starr-Weiner report on sex and sexuality. In: *Mature Years.* New York: McGraw-Hill.

Steinmetz, J., Thompson, L. W., Breckenridge, J., & Gallagher, D. (1985), Behavior group therapy with the elderly: A psychoeducational model. In: *Handbook of Behavioral Group Therapy,* ed. D. Upper & S. Rose. New York: Plenum, pp. 275–302.

Steuer, J. L. & Hammen, C. L. (1983), Cognitive-behavioral group therapy for the depressed elderly: Issues and adaptations. *Cognitive Ther. & Research,* 7:285–296.

────── Mintz, J., Hammen, C. L., Hill, M. A., Jarvik, L. F., McCarley, T., Motoike, P., & Rosen, R. (1984), Cognitive-behavioral and psychodynamic group psychotherapy in treatment of geriatric depression. *J. Consult. & Clin. Psychol.,* 52(4):80–189.

────── ────── Jarvik, L. F. (1982), Geriatric depression: Methodological issues in comparing pharmacology with group psychotherapy results. Conference on psychodynamic research prospectives on development, psychopathology, and treatment in later life. Paper presented at NIMH Center conference on aging, Washington.

Sue, D. W. (1981), *Counseling and the Culturally Different: Theory and Practice.* New York: Wiley.

Sue, S. (1983), Ethnic minority issues in psychology. *Amer. Psychologist,* 38:583–592.

Szapacznik, J., Kurtines, W. M., Santisteban, D., & Perez-Vidal, A. (1982), Ethnic and cultural variations in the care of the aged: New directions in the treatment of depression in the elderly: A life-enhancement counseling approach. *J. Geriatric Psychiat.*, 25:257–281.

Thompson, L. W., Gallagher, D., Nies, G., & Epstein, D. (1983), Evaluation of the effectiveness of professionals and non-professionals as instructors of "coping with depression": Classes for elders. *Gerontologist*, 23:390–396.

Tieberman, M. A., & Guarack, N. (1979), Evaluating the effects of change groups on the elderly. *Internat. J. Group Psychother.*, 29:283–304.

Toseland, R. (1977), Problem-solving group workshop for older persons. *Social Work*, 22:325–326.

Turbow, S. R. (1969), Geriatric group day care and its effect on independent living. *Gerontologist*, 9:508–510.

van der Kolk, A. (1983), The idealizing transference and group psychotherapy with elderly patients. *J. Geriatric Psychiat.*, 16:99–103.

Waters, E., Fink, S., & White, B. (1976), Peer group counseling for older people. *Educational Gerontology*, 1:157–169.

Werbin, J., & Hynes, P. (1979), Transference and culture in a Latino therapy group. *Internat. J. Group Psychother.*, 25:396–401.

White, M. T., & Weiner, M. B. (1986), *The Theory and Practice of Self Psychology*. New York: Brunner/Mazel.

Williams, J. L., Csalany, A., & Misevic, G. (1967), Drug therapy with or without group discussion: Effects on various regimens on the behavior of geriatric patients in a mental hospital. *J. Amer. Geriatrics Soc.*, 15:34–40.

Williams, M., Roback, H., & Pro, J. (1980), A geriatrics "growth group." *Group*, 4(3):43–49.

Wolff, K. (1963), *Geriatric Psychiatry*. Springfield, Ill.: Thomas.

——— (1970), *The Emotional Rehabilitation of the Geriatric Patient*. Springfield, Ill.: Thomas.

Wolk, R. L., & Goldfarb, A. I. (1967), The response to group psychotherapy of aged recent admissions compared with long-term mental hospital patients. *Amer. J. Psychiat.*, 123:10.

Yalom, I. D. (1975), *The Theory and Practice of Group Psychotherapy*. New York: Basic Books.

——— Terrazas, F. (1968), Group therapy for psychotic elderly patients. *Amer. J. Nursing*, 68:1690–1694.

Yesavage, J. A., & Karasu, T. B. (1983), Psychotherapy with elderly patients. *Amer. J. Psychother.*, 36:41–55.

Zimberg, S. (1969), Outpatient geriatric psychiatry in an urban ghetto with non-professional workers. *Amer. J. Psychiat.*, 125:1697–1702.

Zung, W. W. K. (1965), A self-rating depression scale. *Arch. Gen. Psychiat.*, 12:63–70.

Part II
Insight Group Therapy

2

Including the Active Elderly in Group Psychotherapy

ROSALYN BENITEZ-BLOCH, D.S.W.

Prior to the 1970s almost all services, including group therapy, were provided to the more dependent elderly through traditional social agencies or through institutions such as hospitals and homes for the aged. The more active elderly in the community were offered limited, activity-focused programs by church groups and community centers. Legislation, begun with the Older Americans Act of 1965 and continuing, provided an increase of services to the active elderly whose numbers and functioning in the community were greater and more visible.

The major developments that ensued provided a broader continuum of services: meals, transportation, housing, medical screening, peer counseling, and psychotherapy. The Community Mental Health Act included the elderly as a legitimate population for psychotherapeutic services in mental health centers. The visibility of the elderly and services for them grew along with an increase in the numbers of professionals working with the elderly. Aging research and professional training spread from federally funded gerontology centers into the community and from community practice and clinical skills to the center programs. The philosophy of services toward older people in this country was redesigned from being given by the goodhearted but unskilled or the professional in isolated instances to a comprehensive social policy rendered by professionals.

It is characteristic in the United States that most social policies that deal with special populations tend to segregate them. Research might be done on ethnic groups, women, children who are orphaned or poor, educationally special populations, etc. There is some validity for segregation of services in populations that would receive little if they were not separate. This has been true of the aged, especially the frail and dependent. But to segregate the active elderly from other age groups and other ages from the active elderly may not be the most effective choice in all circumstances. It happens that professional segregation of those who work with the elderly also follows. It is not unusual to find an attitude among professionals that those who work with children or younger adults are more sophisticated in their treatment knowledge and skills. The psychoanalytic community was intensely focused on early childhood, expanded to adolescence and adulthood, and only recently has developed a serious therapeutic interest in the elderly. Life cycle curriculum has not included much about the aged, tending to become more involved with death and dying than with living when old. Programs and services are not designed on a life cycle continuum. It is not realistic to expect professionals to learn all skills for all seasons, but it might be more helpful for all populations if there were a less disjunctive perception of the life cycle. Sylvia Plath (1981) expressed the idea in a single poetic line: "In me she has drowned a young girl, and in me an old woman" (p. 38).

GROUP THERAPY

Most of my social work career has been in social agencies as a clinician and administrator, or in universities related to clinical teaching; the last ten years in full-time private practice have enabled me to experience different models of group psychotherapy, including the heterogeneous group. My cotherapist is a psychiatrist who has worked less with older people. We decided to include active older persons in our groups, at first tentatively and then purposely. The term "active" refers to someone living in the community who is relatively independent, relatively healthy, mentally active, and wanting still to uncover, work through, and understand conflicts. We did not include the frail elderly even if mentally alert, nor those with organicity even if this were only occasional, nor the physically ill, nor those with chronic mental illness. The problems of such older people are of a different nature and would complicate and interfere with the work of an "ordinary" group. Homogeneous groups may be more practical and more therapeutic for the aged with such difficulties.

We have found that groups that are heterogeneous both in age and gender can be a benefit for all group members. Conflicts within oneself that relate to various life phases are more accessible when mirrored by a younger person, as are intrafamilial and intergenerational conflicts. The varied transferences provide a wide field for projection, displacement, and triangulation for all members and offer opportunities to work out ambivalence to the other generation, either older or younger. Protectiveness between the generations is more visible in a mixed age group, as is antagonism. Criticism from another group member is easier to hear and consider than it is from one's own mother or daughter. The nurturing that one receives in the group, and the dependency that is allowed, is less conflict-laden than with parents from whom one is trying to separate or come closer. Recently, a thirty-year-old woman was able to reveal in a group session what she had just begun to see as the "crazy" behavior of a parent. The group members helped her work through her feelings of disrespect and disloyalty so that she was able to use the group to reflect her own feelings of "craziness" and separate from them as something that really belonged to her parents. A year later she felt sad that her mother dealt with a situation in such a "crazy" way and was not at that moment aware of how separate she had become.

From an older person's viewpoint there may be cultural values, perhaps old world values, that are rejected by a younger family member, while these may be seen more positively by a group member of the same generation. One group member has repeatedly said to an older woman around this issue, "I really wish you had been my mother." Resolutions that are not possible in a life situation may often be rewoven in group therapy. This is especially true if a parent or a child is already dead. This same idealized mother image in the group was, at another time, able to respond to the younger woman's guilt about leaving home: "You did what was right for you; I should have pushed Lorraine [her own daughter] to become more independent. It would have made her more adult."

The group has a reflective quality that allows members to see what they may become and where they have been. It provides some life cycle integration that is similar to real life, including the experience of death, which may not be the death of the eldest member. Our experience in the psychotherapy group is in contrast to other group experiences, such as those in SAGE (Senior Actualization and Growth Encounter), which seemed to help with marital situations but had not much positive effect on intergenerational strains. Those groups did seem to have good effect as a source of feedback in maintaining the self (Lieberman and Gourash, 1979).

THE SELF AND MIRRORING IN GROUP PSYCHOTHERAPY

Mirroring in group psychotherapy is relevant for the active older person in relation to the sense of self. A part of every problem that an older person brings to group psychotherapy is related to an insult to the sense of self, whether reflective of an internal memory, an interaction, or a physical change. The reality of American culture does not reflect aging as a positive value. The group does reflect each member as unique and valuable, and is symbolic of a society which is therapeutic. Sometimes the search for psychotherapy itself can be an insult, as many psychotherapists do not see older people. Others may see only one or two. Many see older persons as hopeless and beyond therapy. For some older persons there is also the financial insult in searching for psychotherapy. As a practical sidelight, it is possible to integrate some older people in a group with an adjusted fee, if that is needed, without creating a problem for the therapist who is in private practice.

The group members described in this paper range in age from their midtwenties upward; the oldest member was in her eighties. It is easier to include older people in a group if the hours are daytime hours or not too late in the evening (5:00–6:30 P.M.). Some older people have difficulties with transportation but seem to be able to make arrangements. Members do not provide transportation for each other and have no contact outside the group; the separate specialness of the group is thereby retained. In some ways the group does not mirror the outside world at all.

We know from material on infancy and early childhood provided by such researchers as Rene Spitz, John Bowlby, and Margaret Mahler that looking at and being looked back at by one's mother is basic to the development of personality; it is how one finds out who one is and who is the other. As one grows older, behavior is reflected back by the social world, either positively or negatively, as rejection or other critical mirroring that produces unhappy feelings or feelings of depression. As one moves in and out of relationships through life there is a constant shift in the revision of self, sometimes with disappointments and sometimes with fulfillments. It is significant that "reflection" is such an important process in psychotherapy, in which one mirrors one's image and is mirrored by the therapist.

S. H. Foulkes (see Pines, 1982) describes how in group therapy, when numbers of people interact, a mirroring occurs which allows one to see a part of oneself, often a repressed part, reflected by another group member. This helps one to get to know oneself better and to contrast one's own behavior with that of others. The difference, according to Pines (1982), is what carries information. Behavior which is similar may be seen as different when it is observed in another person. Persons may see themselves in the future as older or remember the past as they view similar behavior in younger members. There is no change and no development without difference and the awareness of it.

The heterogeneous group offers life cycle differences that provide mirroring to resolve conflicts that may have roots in one's past, allows for review, and offers an experience that is validating of one's present self. This may be especially important to the older person, who may have neither years nor opportunities available. The problems of older people in group psychotherapy are not different from those of younger people but do have some age-specific aspects: (1) there is more history, more cumulative trauma, more practiced strengths, and less time ahead for testing or resolving in reality; (2) there is often a constricted real life environment due to physical limitations and losses of significant relationships, possessions, and social roles; (3) the group provides for older people an immediate and newly accessible environment when one's world has shrunk and opportunities for new relationships are fewer. The group may become a more intense investment for the older person, a phenomenon we observed in dramatic fashion when a woman drove through a bad storm to come to the group while some of the younger members thought the weather too harsh to battle. She had a heart attack while driving and required hospitalization. She later commented on having had the group to look forward to as part of her recovery goal.

GROUP DYNAMICS

Through two representative group vignettes the reflective and mirroring impact of group members on one another will be illustrated. There are other interactional processes in group psychotherapy that are equally important, but these are intentionally neglected.

Betsy

Betsy is an obese woman, soon to be seventy, a lesbian who has never had a sexual relationship with a man. Her longstanding companion died after a lingering illness during which Betsy took care of her. The group was supportive during this time. After the death of her friend Betsy was left with an abyss in her life—a feeling of having no intimacy and feelings of self-disgust regarding her body. She felt hopeless about any other relationship and saw no future for herself. Earlier losses were brought up: a sister who had died; a brother-in-law who had remarried too quickly; a father who had never accepted her; her having never borne a child; sadness that she had never risked herself with a man. Betsy was envious of women in the group who had heterosexual relationships that provided companionship, and she was disappointed when these relationships seemed less than ideal. One woman in her late twenties responded to Betsy with her own thoughts of having a lesbian relationship to protect herself from the hurts that a man could inflict on her. Together Betsy and Laurie were able to reflect on their fantasies, their fears of closeness, and past disappointments; both were able to see that age was not the issue. The older was able to encourage the younger to take risks, while Laurie was able to offer proof of acceptance to Betsy.

Maria, a young woman of thirty-three, who like Betsy had a weight problem, talked about the isolation she felt because of fears of getting too close to a man. She and Betsy mirrored how each of them built walls of flesh to protect themselves from hurt. The two women, at very different ages, resonated to each other's fixation and regression as they related past disappointments.

Betsy, although the oldest member, was really the baby of the group. Even when someone confronted her with her own denied behavior she was pleased, experiencing it as a form of nurturing and dependency on the group. Laurie and Betsy competed for this role more intensely with the male therapist and became aware of their earlier desires for their own fathers' attention. During one session Laurie became angry with Betsy but was fearful of expressing it. With encouragement, even from Betsy, what emerged was Laurie's being able to say, "I am terrified that I will be like you when I get older, alone, with no friends, feeling sorry for myself." Betsy was the one in the group most empathic with Laurie's feelings, accepting them.

Max

Max was a man of eighty-one, a rather substantial businessman who still ran an enterprise from his home. He had given up his office when his wife, who was younger, developed organic brain syndrome. Her forgetfulness, bizarre dress, inappropriate comments to people, and her hostility to a series of housekeepers kept Max in a constant state of anxiety. He was highly obsessive-compulsive and would not consider placing his wife outside the home. Because of his acute embarrassment about her behavior he withdrew from an active social life in the community. Max had one son, who had had a "nervous breakdown" and who worked with him in the business, although Max did not consider him very competent. A daughter, who was worried about Max, was the source of referral. She was considered the "bad" child by the mother because she had left home, married, and moved away. This was perceived as rejection.

In the group Max was able to vent his anger and disappointment with life with somewhat less guilt than he experienced when alone. Two younger group members mirrored his feelings of embarrassment in relation to parents who were failing and about whom they felt a great sense of burden. The group provided an atmosphere in which feelings, even shameful ones, could be expressed and accepted, without feeling that anyone was harmed. Several group members could relate to Max's frustration with his son and the burdens of children who did not achieve their hopes. One man in his midthirties, who was also in business with a relative, reflected on Max's son with empathy. Nick felt the frustrations of always being the kid and never having the opportunity to be trusted with the role of authority. This gave Max some ideas about the role he assigned his son and allowed Max to give up small responsibilities to him. Younger people in the group experienced their own reflected processes from Max, some needing more separation from parents and others wishing that they could have had the support and protectiveness that Max offered. Symbolically, Max was the clan leader who refused to step down.

The group became Max's new closeness. He would not speak with friends, fearing to be disloyal to his wife, but he could trust this life-removed environment. Max received much encouragement from group members of all ages who could identify with his desire to still enjoy life. He was able to rely more on a housekeeper some days of the week so that he could get out for a few hours to eat with a friend or to attend a meeting. These experiences, along with the group, expanded life for him. Max was able to find, through mirroring by the group, a new value in a sense of self that was different from his past sense of self, which had been more dependent on work and financial worth. He was able to respond to group members with more feeling and with less need to be the authority. When a younger member of the group died, Max was able to accept the comfort of the group and allowed members to relieve him of guilt because he was older and still alive.

When the group is confronted with death, there is a loosening of defenses and painful material is resonated. The experience of losing a group member through death may help to experience the work of mourning. For those who remain, there is the realization that, although invisible in the group, the lost member is still important, mentioned from time to time because of a recalled comment or a way of coping. Older members know that, if they should die while in the group, they too will be remembered and that group members will not run from the mourning experience. A group sense of ongoing experience may be analogous to the experience of the individual self.

LIMITATIONS

It is not always possible to arrange one's practice to include different generations in a group. The experienced therapist will be flexible and have both heterogeneous and homogeneous groups, depending on circumstances. When heterogeneous groups as described in this chapter are not possible, the therapist, who is usually younger, can foster an environment that provokes an age consciousness that allows some of the same conflicts to emerge. The skills of the therapist and the therapist's own resolution of intergenerational issues are important influences in all groups that deal with intergenerational feelings, whether in homogeneous or heterogeneous groups. Both types of group can be of help in working through life cycle experiences for the growth of the therapist as well as for group members.

CONCLUSION

If various generations are represented in a group the sense of self is expanded. The group is all generations and is experienced by each member in this way. Experiencing oneself in a life cycle process becomes more imaginable, as does the resolution of intergenerational issues. This kind of heterogeneous group including active older persons avoids unnecessary segregation for both the old and the younger members. It reflects a less disjunctive perception of the span of life.

REFERENCES

Lieberman, M., & Gourash, N. (1979), Evaluating the effects of change groups on the elderly. *Internat. J. Group Psychother.*, 29:283–304.
Pines, M. (1982), Reflections on mirroring. *Group Analysis*, 15:1–24.
Plath, S. (1981), *Collected Poems.* London: Faber & Faber.

3

Group Therapies with the Elderly: Issues and Prospects

MARTIN LAKIN, Ph.D.

Old age in the United States is characterized by the interrelated conditions of decreased social interactions, lowered income, declining health, limited housing options, a narrowing circle of friends of one's own age, and an increasing incidence of widowhood. Retirement presents a major life crisis to many persons, particularly males, as in our present industrial society the old are judged, and tend to judge themselves, against the standards set by those who work. Social class characteristics of those over sixty-five tend to compound these typical life circumstances, since the aged have typically been more poorly educated than younger persons.

Compared to younger persons, those over sixty-five show higher rates of psychopathology in general, depression in particular. Despite this disproportionate need, statistics for institutions, community mental health centers, and private practice all show an underutilization of mental health services by those over sixty-five (Group for the Advancement of Psychiatry, 1970; Blank, 1974; Kahn, 1975). The dismal status of mental health care delivery for the aged has been known for a long time. According to the Group for the Advancement of Psychiatry report of over a decade ago, "Older patients do not receive early and adequate care in the community but tend to be institutionalized in mental hospitals, nursing homes, and other care facilities with little likelihood of discharge . . . the elderly suffer disproportionately from our non-system of non-care, characterized by insufficient financing for both health and sickness and by fragmented delivery of services" (p. 657).

ATTITUDES OF PSYCHOTHERAPISTS

One of the reasons for inadequate psychological services for the elderly is the mutually negativistic attitudes toward gerontological psychotherapy held by the aged themselves and by the mental health professionals who might treat them. Underlying these attitudes is a pervasive prejudice against the aged, termed "ageism" by Butler (1975): "Ageism allows those of us who are younger to see old people as 'different.' We subtly cease to identify with them as human beings, which enables us to feel more comfortable about our neglect and dislike of them. . . . Ageism is a thinly disguised attempt to avoid the personal reality of human aging and death" (p. 894).

For the psychotherapist, the aspect of ageism that involves seeing the aged as "different" takes the form of a widely shared assumption that the aged are rigid and cannot voluntarily change themselves psychologically. Calls for more extensive therapeutic efforts with the elderly have blamed current biases on this shared pessimism about the abilities of older individuals to benefit from psychotherapies, particularly those which attempt to resolve inner conflict or foster an awareness of ambivalent feelings. With the possible exception of Jung's ideas, theories of psychotherapy seem to have been fashioned mainly for the problems of young and early adulthood. Obstacles to self-fulfillment in early to middle life stages are accentuated. There is a focus on developmental guilt, sexual anxieties, and on the inhibitions and insecurities which prevent full adult achievement rather than on coping with inevitable decline, or finding new interests and goals as one becomes old.

RESEARCH ON PSYCHOLOGICAL IMPAIRMENT

The lack of resolution about the extent of physiological, cognitive, and emotional impairments in the aged, as well as the sources of these limitations, has been a persistent theme in the literature on psychotherapy with the aged (see Rechtschaffen, 1959). Even though recent research might be viewed as debunking the stereotyped image of the elderly as grossly impaired in terms of basic psychological functioning, the images of limitations associated with it persist. But studies by Palmore (1970), Granick and Patterson (1971), and Schaie (1974), have cast doubt on the generality of cognitive decline with age, and there is evidence that much of the observed decline in cognitive ability is attributable to specific diseases or disabilities rather than to the aging process per se. Some mental disabilities one sees among the aged may be secondary to, or contingent upon, impairments involving the vital contact areas of vision and hearing. Were the physical illnesses treated and the sensory impairments compensated for, so the argument goes, the elderly would be more suitable candidates for psychotherapy, much as younger persons.

While physically healthy elderly persons do show an overall reduced speed in reacting to stimuli and increased time taken for information processing, Fozard and Thomas (1975) point out that age alone is a very weak predictor of personality or behavior. Indeed, Grotjahn (1955) argues that resistance against unpleasant insights is *lessened* in old age and character defenses have in many cases softened rather than hardened because of the confrontation of realistic changes. Thus, Neugarten (1970) describes a great variety of adaptations to aging and provides a basis for distinctions between the "young-old" (sixty-five to seventy-five) and the "old-old" (seventy-five plus). A problem with much of the research which is limitation-focused is that it has been done on the disabled, the institutionalized, or the debilitated, i.e., the confused or demented. Rigidity and flexibility are not age but personality variables according to Kahana (1979).

We see that research evidence does not support the argument that gross decline in cognitive abilities and emotional expressiveness with old age is inevitable, or that it makes the elderly unsuitable candidates for psychotherapy. However, people's tendency to believe in this argument has an important impact on their behavior toward the elderly. Clearly, the level of communication between therapist and the elderly client will be less than optimal, to the extent that the therapist erroneously considers—consciously or unconsciously—all old people to be impaired.

Do these considerations imply that the elderly may be treated in therapies, particularly group therapies, just like younger adults? I will present some research data which suggests that accommodation of group techniques to the elderly is necessary, but this may be necessitated by cultural rather than biological differences. Lawton (1976) states that certain traits commonly found among elderly persons in our culture do indeed mandate different psychological intervention strategies with them. They are the following:

1. The elderly are, on average, less educated—and thus considerably less familiar with psychological ideas and terminology—than are younger individuals.

2. Many elderly persons reject and resist the implicit moral relativism and the liberal ideologies which characterize contemporary psychotherapies.

3. Psychological concepts, terminology, and descriptions of behavior are foreign and vaguely threatening to many elderly individuals.

4. Older persons are characteristically reluctant to admit a need for psychological assistance, deeming such admission tantamount to acknowledging personal "craziness."

Kahana (1979) takes the position that in the light of such characteristics a psychotherapist must be more careful in choosing terms, and cautious in pushing patients to explore the sources of troubled or conflicted inner feelings and ambivalent relationships. One cannot rely upon metaphorical abstractions or generalizations, but must be prepared for a more concrete as well as a somewhat slower pace of therapy interaction. One must certainly not assume a familiarity with psychodynamic interpretation methods.

ADAPTATION OF THERAPY TECHNIQUES FOR THE ELDERLY CLIENT

Many psychotherapists recommend accommodation to physical and psychological limitations of the elderly by means of shorter but more frequent sessions. For example, in adapting insight therapy for use with the aged, Lewis and Butler (1974) urge the use of the elderly's compulsion to reminisce as a form of "free association," while Weinberg (1957) suggests exploiting two characteristics of the elderly as clients: their eagerness to follow directions and their capacity for the delay of gratification. Others (e.g., Ross, 1959) report successful use of dual therapists, refreshments, music, and even group singing and dancing as a warm-up before group therapy sessions. However, most workers with the aged agree that compared to therapy with younger clients, gerontological psychotherapy usually requires a more active role on the part of the therapist. It also requires a more explicit indication of the boundaries of what the therapist can and will do.

In a study of age differences in the perception of a therapy relationship (Kowal, Kemp, Lakin, and Wilson, 1964), young, middle-aged, and elderly males and females were shown TAT-type drawings of a therapy consulting room scene. The ages of depicted "clients" and "therapists" paralleled the ages of the groups of subjects. The scenes were defined as follows: "A person is seeking psychological help from this expert about his/her personal problems." In the stories elicited, aged and middle-aged persons attributed less readiness for self-disclosure and self-exploration than did younger persons. Similarly, the two older groups tended to disavow personal responsibility for problems more than did the younger persons. On the other hand, while perhaps less "open" than young adults, the old people were as open as the middle-aged.

A marked age differential between therapist and client may present difficulties for both parties. In general, age comparisons figure prominently in what the analytically oriented would call transference reactions. Actually, such reactions are ubiquitous though differently utilized (or ignored) depending on the therapy technique. The therapist may be seen as parent surrogate or as child surrogate, and the client's perception of these "transferred" attributes arouse corresponding ambivalences, dependency, and anxieties. The elderly may be skeptical of a younger person's ability to empathize with the fears and concerns of an older person. The earlier discussion of ageism suggests that this skepticism may to a considerable extent be warranted. Certainly it helps if therapists are themselves older, or have good training in geropsychology that enriches their understanding of, and ability to deal with, problems faced by the aged.

CONSIDERATIONS OF GROUP THERAPY WITH THE ELDERLY

Individual therapy is generally preferable to group therapy for those elderly clients who require a great deal of personal support, who are excessively fearful or paranoid, or for those whose communication abilities are greatly impaired. It is harder to apply the supportive "shoring up" of a person in the face of the undeniable stresses of a group situation than it is to be supportive in the more controllable dyadic arrangement.

Experience in psychotherapy with the aged, however, suggests that group may provide the benefits of a social context as well as economical therapeutic services. The therapy group can be responsive to the fact of frequent isolation among the aged. Many group therapists conceive of the group as a symbolically recreated familial experience and see the individual in it as "working through" basic emotional problems in an emotionally corrective setting. Reports have noted that elderly group participants also tend to show reversals in general deterioration, including improvement in personal hygiene and appearance (Ross, 1959), noticeable improvement in social interest and mental functioning (Kubie and Landau, 1953), and improved interpersonal relationships (Wolff, 1967). These reported benefits are consistent with the position that continued social involvement, at least of this special type, is beneficial for the morale of old people. The multiperson context also stimulates mutual comparisons and elicits support in the face of what comes to be perceived as common or shared concerns. This sharing of problems is especially useful for the elderly, as they so frequently have to cope with disability, loss, and death.

On the other hand, several features of group therapies pose special problems for older people. For example, a typical initial reaction to group therapy at any age is ambivalence, but for older people fear of status devaluation compounds this ambivalence. The frightening vulnerability attached to disclosing inner feelings to a group can overshadow the implicit promise of support and encouragement. The fear of disclosure can be intensified by the possibility of lowered self-esteem as a consequence. The reluctance of older people to disclose might be especially great in a multi-age group, due to the absence of peers who might be viewed as potentially more understanding than younger persons. However, Kahana and Kahana (1970a, 1970b) report that mixing old and young on the same ward will result in improved cognitive function in the older patient. Butler (1975) also maintains that older people can benefit from multi-age groups. On the other hand, a "we-they" posture can be collectively established only by homogeneous group participants. As members of a disadvantaged minority, the elderly in a homogeneous group can commiserate and gain mutual support as elderly persons. The age-segregated group's obvious benefits of mutual support should be weighed against the possible advantages of multi-age groups.

COMPARING OLD AND YOUNG IN GROUPS

In recent years there has been a marked increase in the use of groups among the elderly for supportive, therapeutic, or recreational purposes (Klein, LeShan, and Furman, 1965; Butler, 1975). However, group workers differ considerably in their ideas of how to use group interventions with this age group. Aside from the ageist bias referred to earlier, questions persist regarding age-associated limitations in terms of capacities for therapeutic interaction with peers. Thus, despite his acknowledged leadership in group work with the aged, Goldfarb offers a conservative assessment: "Younger persons in group psychotherapy break, remake, test, and consolidate relationship with others and . . . acquire insights. [However], older people do not seem to go through this process in their groups, no matter what the interests or the skills of the therapist" (in Klein, LeShan, and Furman, 1965, p. 12).

To this point I have considered both sides of the "suitability for psychotherapy" issue, and have suggested that group therapy can be an appropriate therapeutic vehicle for the elderly *provided* the group intervention takes into account the special characteristics of the elderly population subset it addresses. To amplify this point I will report a study I recently conducted with two graduate students. While it does not use a formal group therapy format, and its participants are not acknowledged psychotherapy patients, I believe it provides indirect confirmation for the need to adapt group therapies for the needs of elderly participants. The study involved a comparison of nonpatient older and younger adults in what we called "discussion" rather than therapy groups because we wanted to study nonpathological samples of group behavior. Believing that the question of realistic goals for the elderly could be studied only by comparative examination of naturally occurring and normative processes in groups of old and young, my coinvestigators and I compared group interactions in five groups of senior citizens (age sixty-five to eighty) and three groups of young adults (age eighteen to twenty-two).[1]

The following group process dimensions derived from Lakin, Lakin, and Costanzo's (1979) study of young children's group behavior were adapted to described discussion-support groups for older and younger adults:

1. *Boundary behaviors* are utterances that indicate group belonging, or "we/they" attributes. Examples are "we old folk," "the young people nowadays," "us senior citizens."

2. *Subgrouping* is coded when there is a "teaming up" of three or more members, usually in solidarity vis-à-vis a position, but also against an individual or another subgroup.

3. *Normative behaviors* include rule making, evaluations of others,

[1]Readers who wish to receive a complete research report may write to the author at the Department of Psychology, Duke University, Durham, NC 27706.

and prescriptive statements (as in "shoulds" and "shouldn'ts") and group standards of behavior.

4. *Organization behaviors* include attempts to lead, changes of focus or direction, and attempts to assign roles or functions to others, or to assume a chairperson role.

5. *Establishing personal significance* includes bids for recognition. It is coded whenever one boasts or brags (i.e., recounts personal achievements or cites family status) or claims attention for a personal attribute, skill, or possession.

6. *Self-disclosure* is sharing inner feelings, intimate personal experiences, or problems not ordinarily told to strangers, and which characteristically involve anhedonic elements, such as losses or personal vulnerabilities.

7. *Conflict behaviors* include disagreements or quarrels that arise in sessions, whether they be mild differences of opinion or emphatic efforts to vanquish opponents.

8. *Support behaviors* are verbalized sympathetic or empathetic utterances in the form of agreements with other members or emotional support for them.

9. *Group to leader* is coded for questions or requests for direction. It may be taken to indicate relative group autonomy or degree of dependence on the leader.

10. *Leader to group* is coded whenever the leader intervenes to ask a question or to suggest a direction for discussion.

11. *Group tone* refers to the emotional atmosphere of the group at any particular point and includes three subscales as follows: (a) light to heavy; (b) comfortable to anxious; (c) attentive to bored.

The groups of the elderly were conducted by the author and the groups of young adults by his graduate assistant, as we wished to maintain relative age similarity between leader and members. The leaders attempted to be as nondirective as possible and intervened only to facilitate the flow of discussion. We began each group with the following explanation of our aim: "Group therapy is currently widely used. We don't know if talking together helps or not, so we are studying the queston by observing folks at *your* time of life talking together. We are interested in seeing how you relate to one another, and we also want to hear about your concerns as well as your satisfactions at *your* time of life." All of the groups met for one hour per week over a seven-week period. Average attendance at group sessions was eight members.

There were significant differences (p < .01) between older adults and the young adults in the following group process dimensions: Boundary, Leader to Group, Self-Disclosure, and Conflict Behaviors, and in one subcategory of Group Tone, i.e., Boredom. Of these dimensions, the first four were significantly higher for all the older groups. That is, elderly group members made more references to differences between themselves and others, demanded and received more leader guidance, disclosed more intimate details to one another, but also fought more among themselves than did young persons. Boredom was significantly higher among young adults. Leader to Group communications were most frequent among the less educated elderly, whereas the more highly educated elderly did not differ from the younger subjects in this respect, i.e., the more educated elderly asked for less leader guidance than did the less educated.

In all the groups of the elderly there was a virtually continuous flow from self-disclosure to reassurance or advice; and almost tranquil sharing followed by seemingly automatic comforting responses. By contrast, in the young adults' group there was a tense or "uptight" quality evidenced by many anxious pauses during sessions. Compared to the young, all the older adults talked with relative ease and, at least initially, virtually no hesitation, about such profound human experiences as loneliness, fears of abandonment, problems of widowhood, and feelings of rejection and vulnerability in the face of apparent indifference in the environment. On the other hand, the responses to such disclosures from peers were somewhat empathic, but almost stereotypic, as if everyone should expect to experience such losses. By comparison, young adults disclosed much less, but when they did they elicited more intense responses from the other members. For instance, when a student would hesitantly express the fear that he couldn't "make it," it would evoke similar apprehensions, revealing much shared anxiety, in contrast to the almost unruffled reactions to self-disclosure in groups of the elderly.

Our speculations were that persons are more likely to openly compare life experiences when they already agree implicitly about the meanings of such experience. The elderly reveal feelings about losses or other age-related concerns with relative confidence that others in the group probably feel the same way. The confidence that others have similar problems facilitates emotional communication (Dickoff and Lakin, 1963). The belief among the old that their problems are shared ones facilitates disclosure, which in turn reinforces the idea that they are not unique in their misfortunes. By contrast, the young believe that they are more alone than they really are, and this in turn inhibits self-disclosure.

What are the implications of the muted emotional tone in the elderly helping groups? I suggest that therapist or group strategies designed to confront, to elicit evidence of intrapsychic and interpersonal tensions, and to insist on the preeminence of here-and-now interactions probably run counter to tendencies among many in this age group to try to lessen the intensity of their emotional reactions. Elderly persons may be more self-protective in the sense that they avoid strong overt reactions to other members. Although such leader strategies are frequently quite useful in helping groups composed of young adults, they are probably less so with groups of the elderly. Group interventions among the elderly should emphasize an accepting, encouraging, supportive, and nonconfrontational mode. They should mainly invite identification with the problems of others through encouragement of sharing and comparing, and avoid attempts to arouse emotional responses.

SOME SUGGESTIONS FOR GROUP WORK WITH THE ELDERLY

I suggest that the group therapist working with the aged emphasize that it is helpful to share and compare, not only in terms of common concerns but also in the pleasures and satisfactions that are common to members of this age group. I consider it important for group workers to carefully weigh their preferred methods of probing, sharing and comparing, and giving and receiving both support and feedback, and to consider these in the light of the operation of security systems among the specific population of the elderly they are working with. In our groups, it was clear that the older participants preferred to talk about concrete issues, such as personal isolation, financial difficulties, the experience of bereavement, or the disadvantaged status of the aged as a class. In contrast to the procedures of many contemporary group therapies, here-and-now issues were ignored, and the idea of analyzing one's own interactions with other group members was regarded as irrelevant.

Even though older adults are likely to share a range of common life experiences, leaders should be aware that older adults are also particularly sensitive to being "lumped together"—because they themselves share common negative stereotypes about aging. In order to work effectively with them, leaders should be prepared to challenge these stereotypes, as well as the commonly held conviction regarding inevitable senility. In this connection, group discussions among elderly persons often take the form of mutual denigration (e.g., "Oh well, he is just another complainer—like most old people are!"). The self-contempt of many older persons tends to generate contemptuous attitudes toward their peers. Shared ideas about positive aspects of aging—maturity, personal development, and spiritual growth—are not common convictions among this age group. In our era of rapid social and technological changes, the wisdom of the elderly is no longer taken for granted, even by the elderly themselves.

To counter the negative view of old age as a useless time of life, group discussion may consider alternative activities, lifestyles, and interests. For instance, one self-help organization, SAGE (Senior Actualization and Growth Exploration), emphasizes this approach, arguing that older people's attitudes toward themselves shape their lives, even affecting their physical well-being. Members are encouraged to be supportive of one another, to maintain contacts beyond the weekly group meetings, and to try out ideas and activities suggested during group interactions.

Because of the heightened concerns of older help seekers about being thought "crazy," it is especially important to avoid the inclusion of grossly disorganized elderly persons with relatively well-functioning ones. Group interventions should also take into account the possibilities of impaired vision or hearing and try to compensate for them in the physical arrangements of the group. While the degree and type of structuring required will vary with the level of functioning, education, and psychological-mindedness of the participants, the leader should be prepared to provide more of it for a group of the elderly. Structural ambiguity that can be relatively productive in dynamically oriented groups of younger adults may be counterproductive and frustrating in groups of the elderly. Intermember tolerance is usually more limited in this age group. For this reason, and because supportive but critical feedback by others is not as easily mobilized to counter persistent and insensitive talkers, it is especially important to prevent monopolization of sessions by long-winded members and to structure "air time" and "equal time" for everyone.

SUMMARY

In this chapter I have attempted to consider the questions posed by therapists and researchers regarding the supposed psychological handicap of elderly persons which would preclude treating them psychotherapeutically. Such handicaps can be especially significant in group therapies. Evidence for theories of psychological limitation would not justify the conclusion that group treatment is inappropriate for the elderly. On the other hand, cohort and culture are to some extent predictors of commonly shared characteristics among elderly persons and do mandate the adaptation of group therapy intervention strategies to meet the needs of the particular subset of elderly being addressed. Some research evidence is introduced to suggest how this might be accomplished.

REFERENCES

Blank, M. L. (1974), Raising the age barrier to psychotherapy. *Geriatrics*, 29:141–148.

Butler, R. N. (1975), Psychiatry and the elderly: An overview. *Amer. J. Psychiat.*, 132:893–900.

Dickoff, H., & Lakin, M. (1963), Patients' views of group psychotherapy: Retrospection and interpretations. *Internat. J. Group Psychother.*, 13:61–73.

Fozard, J. L., & Thomas, J. C., Jr. (1975), Psychology of aging: Basic factors and some psychiatric applications. In: *Modern Perspectives in the Psychiatry of Old Age*, ed. J. G. Howells. New York: Brunner/Mazel, pp. 107–169.

Granick, S., & Patterson, R. D. (1971), *Human Aging: II. An Eleven-Year Biomedical and Behavioral Study*. Public Health Service Monograph 71–9037. Washington, D.C.: U.S. Government Printing Office.

Grotjahn, M. (1955), Analytic psychotherapy with the elderly. *Psychoanal. Rev.*, 42:419–427.

Group for the Advancement of Psychiatry (1970), *Toward a Public Policy on Mental Health Care of the Elderly*. Vol. VII, Report No. 79.

Jourard, S. M. (1971), *Self-disclosure: An Experimental Analysis of the Transparent Self*. New York: Wiley.

Kahana, B., & Kahana, E. (1970a), Changes in mental status of elderly patients in age-integrated and age-segregated hospital milieus. *J. Abnorm. Psychol.*, 25:177–181.

Kahana, E., & Kahana, B. (1970b), Therapeutic potential of age-integration: Effects of age-integrated environments on elderly psychiatric patients. *Arch. Gen. Psychiat.*, 23:20–29.

Kahana, R. J. (1979), Psychodynamic psychotherapy with the aged. *J. Geriatric Psychiat.*, 12:71–100.

Kahn, R. L. (1975), The mental health system and the future aged. *Gerontologist*, 15:24–31.

Klein, W. H., LeShan, E. J., & Furman, S. S. (1965), *Promoting Mental Health of Older People Through Group Methods: A Practical Guide*. New York: Mental Health Materials Center.

Kowal, K., Kemp, D. E., Lakin, M., & Wilson, S. (1964), Perception of the helping relationship as a function of age. *J. Gerontol.*, 19:405–413.

Kubie, S. H., & Landau, G. (1953), *Group Work with the Aged*. New York: International Universities Press.

Lakin, M., Lakin, M., & Costanzo, P. (1979), Group processes in early child-hood: A dimension of human development. *Internat. J. Behav. Devel.* 2:171–183.

Lawton, M. P. (1976), Geropsychological knowledge as a background for psychotherapy with older people. *J. Geriatric Psychiat.*, 9:221–234.

Lewis, M. I., & Butler, R. N. (1974), Life review therapy: Putting memories to work. *Geriatrics*, 29:165–173.

McGee, J., & Lakin, M. (1977), Social perspectives on psychotherapy with the aged. *Psychotherapy: Theory, Research & Practice*, 14:333–342.

Neugarten, B. L. (1970), Dynamics of transitions of middle age to old age: Adaptation and the life cycle. *J. Geriatric Psychiat.*, 4:71–87.

Palmore, E., Ed. (1970), *Normal Aging I*. Durham: Duke University Press.

Rechtschaffen, A. (1959), Psychotherapy with geriatric patients: A review of the literature. *J. Gerontol.*, 14:73–84.

Ross, M. (1959), Recent contributions to gerontologic group psychotherapy. *Internat. J. Group Psychother.*, 9:442–450.

Schaie, K. W. (1974), Translations in gerontology—from lab to life: Intellectual functioning. *Amer. Psychologist*, 29:802–807.

Weinberg, J. (1957), Psychotherapy of the aged. In: *Progress in Psychotherapy*, ed. J. H. Masserman. New York: Grune & Stratton.

Wolff, K. (1967), Comparison of group and individual psychotherapy with geriatric patients. *Dis. Nerv. Syst.*, 28:384–386.

4

The Third Chance: Self Psychology as an Effective Group Approach for Older Adults

MARCELLA BAKUR WEINER, Ed.D. and MARJORIE TAGGART WHITE, Ph.D.

Louise, a community-living older woman in her seventies, is in a group therapy session. She is telling the group how distressed she is living with her husband who, suffering some form of senility, no longer responds to her. "He is," she says, "empty and far-away; I feel as though he is constantly turning away from me, even though I understand he can't help it."

Alice, another group member of similar age, turns to Louise and gently says, "You know, I really feel for you. It must be awful. It reminds me of the incident you told us about when you first came into the group. Remember, when you were four and first met your new stepmother?" Louise catches Alice's eye and nods in appreciation as her eyes fill with tears. The incident Alice is referring to happened to Louise when she was four. Her mother had died over a year before, and her father was about to remarry. He announced to his four-year-old that she was to have a new Mommy, whom she would now meet. A strange woman came into the room. Full of anticipation and excitement, the little Louise ran toward her exclaiming, "Momma, Momma, look how high I can jump!" and proceeded to jump up and down in self-display. The new lady turned to her, saying, "Don't call me Momma. Call me Auntie!" and walked away. Seventy years later Louise still remembers the event and how hurt she had felt. Now part of a group, she has shared the experience with others, who, as Alice had, empathized with her and made her feel understood. These others, and the leader, a trained clinician, are new "selfobjects," and the group approach is called self psychology. In this context Louise, and others in later life, experience soothing and reparation, a way of healing early wounds. Hope for more joyful, satisfying living is offered as a possibility, regardless of age.

The "third chance" offered Louise and other group members reflects the approach of the late Heinz Kohut's self psychology. Within this framework, the group therapy experience offers three major selfobject transferences: mirror, idealizing, and twinship transferences. Aspects of the twinship need were evident in the relationship between Louise and Alice, who had found each other and formed an alliance based on their perceived overall likeness. With both Louise and Alice, early development had been insufficient in promoting healthy mirroring and idealizing. Instead, the group now provided an arena for the formation of the twinship and for the belated fulfillment of earlier needs for self-validation. This twinship or alter ego selfobject need was seen by Kohut (1984) as involving a deep human need to share similar feelings and experiences with people like oneself: "There are still people who derive the sustenance that maintains their selves mainly from feeling surrounded by alter egos. They feel strong and cohesive as members of a group of people whom they experience as being in essence like them, doing similar work, sharing similar biases and predilections, and the like" (p. 203). In stressing the human quality of the twinship selfobject need—to feel human among human beings—Kohut predicts that these feelings may in turn be a bridge to object love. The union between Louise and Alice, though both were of advanced age, had the caring quality, in a sensitivity to what the other person feels and thinks (although the other may not be experienced at a deep level as having an independent center of initiative), that may lead, if it is desired, to romantic love.

With Louise, both early mirroring (the first chance) and idealization possibilities (the second) were unrealized, and psychological scars rendered her aging highly vulnerable to narcissistic onslaughts. This was evidenced by her hypochondriacal symptoms and frequent complaining in the group. Perceiving her early world as nonresponsive, she was reacting to it with complaints. Since confrontation was never employed by the leader, in accordance with her approach, interpretations of an empathic nature (e.g., "I can understand that you would feel this way given your sense of how unfairly you have been treated") were offered instead. The leader thus offered herself as a model for reparative soothing, which the other group members reflected. This approach stands in contrast to group experiences that are structured to be stressful, in which persons report feeling "attacked" by the group and "unprotected" by the leader. In the context of the authors' approach, the existence of such feelings would be interpreted as a sign of empathic failure.

THE EMPATHIC STANCE AND THE ENCOURAGEMENT OF HEALTHY NARCISSISM

Marie was reluctant to join a group. Sixty-eight, active, and healthy, she had sought individual therapy for depression and vaguely defined feelings of anxiety. Her individual therapist, whom she had seen a few times, suggested group. Hesitatingly, she joined. After a few sessions, she left, horrified. In the new group, she is recounting her experiences in the previous one. Early in life Marie had had a bout with polio. This left her with a slight limp and a problem buying shoes that would fit her and reduce the limp. Always dressing well and taking evident pride in this, she sometimes spent hours searching for shoes. She had spoken of this in her former group, spelling out her difficulties. Dr. J., the group leader, had asked her why she did not have special shoes made. Marie had told the group and the therapist: "But I spent years as a child wearing just that kind of awful-looking shoe and waiting for kids to ask me why I was wearing those 'old lady' shoes! Sometimes, they would just point and whisper. When they laughed, it was the worst! I want to forget all those awful years and how hard I fought to learn to buy regular shoes and look like everyone else." To Marie's horror, she heard the group therapist say: "If only you weren't so vain!" Marie said she started to cry, as though at sixty-eight she were again reliving all the pain of those early years. She went home and never returned to the group.

In her new group, the leader and members were empathizing with murmurs of "I can understand how you felt!" and "Why shouldn't you want to look attractive?" The group therapist, using self psychology, realized that it was not so much the previous therapist's failure to tune in on her childhood suffering as it was his flagrant disapproval of her "vanity" that had made Marie feel completely uncared for. To imply that she was pathologically narcissistic in her natural desire to be admired and thought attractive "like everyone else" was to deny her inborn need and right to be exhibitionistic, as if her childhood handicap had permanently deprived her of the appreciative mirroring she so desperately needed to compensate for her childhood traumas. Fortunately, Marie's childhood experiences seemed to have given her enough healthy mirroring and ambition to strive to overcome her handicap and make the most of her assets. Yet her self-esteem was dangerously vulnerable, not only because of the polio trauma but also because her father had suddenly disappeared in an impetuous separation from her mother.

Her expectations that an empathic father figure would be reliably available to her had been severely undermined by her father's disappearance. This had made it difficult for her to trust other men to be dependably loving. At sixty-eight, though she had entered a number of relationships with men, none were of a lasting nature. Holding the unconscious conviction that her childhood problems had driven her father away, she continued to discourage other men. She was at first easily convinced that what she experienced as the remoteness and insensitivity of Dr. J. was all she, poor maimed Marie, could ever expect—unless she became what Dr. J. and other "acceptable" men expected her to be, whatever mysterious way of being that was. But Dr. J.'s judgmental "maturity morality," his criticizing her for her "vanity" when she was struggling so hard to compensate for her handicap, made her suddenly realize that the gap in understanding between this therapist and her feelings was too huge. Whatever he wanted to develop her into she wouldn't want to be, at sixty-eight or any age.

Marie stayed in the new group and in individual treatment for several years. The therapist's empathy and that of the group helped her develop further into a warm, sexually interested, and self-confident woman. Empathy, a necessary vehicle for "cure," is an essential element of self psychology; it is the unique human capacity to feel oneself into another's psychological life, to understand it, and, on the basis of that understanding, to provide a "powerful emotional bond between people" (White, 1984, p. 16). It is the attempt to participate in the other's psychological life as a development-enhancing selfobject, to compensate for the inadequacies of the original parental selfobject.

THE DEVELOPMENT OF A COHESIVE SELF

It is sometimes hard to remember that the patient sitting before us in individual or group settings, who is now of advanced age, was once a child. But of course that is so, and consequently the complex patterns that now appear have taken many years to form. Self psychology focuses on the development of a cohesive, harmonious self. Self psychologists propose that the Oedipus complex can be a joyful experience and can lead to normal, happy sexuality when the child, and the child's competitive sexuality, are accepted in a nonpathological environment. Proper development, allowing a concentration on the self, should lead to the normal "healthy narcissism or self-love of the well-mothered infant" (Grotjahn, 1981, p. 14). Conversely, the self's inadequate development in reaction to an unresponsive environment is the reason for narcissistic disturbance, a fragile self tending easily toward self-fragmentation when the environment is perceived as nonresponsive. The role of both the group therapist and the group members is to cement a fractured self, creating one that is healthy and whole. Healthy development of the nuclear self is fostered by the selfobject relationships that can develop between the child and his parents, relationships that are essential to growth.

GROUP AND THE OLDER ADULT: THE ROLE OF THE THERAPIST

Before introducing the older patient into the group, whether age-homogeneous or age-heterogeneous, the therapist works with the patient in preparatory individual sessions, the object being to establish a "firm selfobject transference" (Harwood, 1983). Once this is accomplished, joining the group, as we have shown, provides the patient a wealth of potential selfobjects: the group's individual members, the therapist, and the group itself. If all goes well, the patient gains the group's acceptance and understanding and draws from its strength, while recognizing the group's separateness and the uniqueness of each individual member. In the group patients can receive empathic understanding, achieve insight into the roots of their problems, and experience empathy with other people.

Though Kohut does not address group therapy in detail, he does state that group pressure may diminish individuality and that the therapist must safeguard the evolving nuclear self. This is done by the therapist's ensuring that all persons are encouraged to discover themselves and to march to the beat of their own drum.

As therapists we are aware that the human mind is not a thing but a group of images, i.e., self- and object representations, which originally represented mother, father, brother, sister, stranger, friends. All are to be eventually perceived, in the natural process of growth, as different from the self. Where there is a lack of a firm self, others are experienced as similar to or as part of the self. Thus, while the "group self" may be clinically expressed in group cohesion, it also offers the older group member the continued possibility for further structural change with respect to individuation. Group therapy per se can stimulate and encourage such individual differentiation as the group itself goes from one stage to another over a period of time.

The therapist plays an essential role in the group setting with older adults. For one, the analyst becomes a selfobject for the patient, "enabling a mirroring or idealizing transference to evolve" (Schwartz-man, 1984a, p. 6). In the mirroring transference the patient maintains self-cohesion through the mirroring of his archaic omnipotent wishful self, while in the idealizing transference it is maintained through merger with the analyst as an idealized parent imago. These two types of transference enable the patient to use the therapist as a selfobject. In turn, this process serves as precursor for the formation of psychic structure through the internalization of good selfobjects. Eventually the use of the therapist as a selfobject comes to include an awareness of the analyst as a separate, whole, and differentiated person, an independent center of initiative (Kohut, 1971).

THE DEVELOPMENT OF A COHESIVE SELF AND GROUP TERMINATION

With the eventual development of a firm, cohesive self, other benefits accrue. The possibility for altruism opens up, as well as feelings of universality—the understanding and acknowledgment that one is not alone in needing affirmation of the grandiose self and merger with an idealized parental imago. Through all this is the strong thread or lifeline of the therapeutic experience as a reworking or redirecting of derailed development in healthier, more rewarding directions.

With the termination of the group experience, the patient's formerly devitalized self has looked to the group and to the therapist whose ideals are admired and whose strength the self can eventually attain. Harwood (1983), describing the process of termination using a self psychology stance, writes:

In the group, if the needs of the nuclear self are allowed to emerge in crystallizing its ambitions under the tract of the grandiose self without severe frustration and to feel stronger under the umbrella of the group idealized parent imago, then, in addition to the attainment of psychic structure, a new, more cohesive self can emerge. This self should then be able to maintain and regulate its own self esteem and retain its ideals while working to realize its ambitions. The group and the therapist will no longer be needed, since their functions will by now be internalized and the patient should be able to terminate with an appreciation of each member's individuality, strengths, and weaknesses. [p. 485]

THE GROUP SELF APPROACH AS DIFFERENT

Consistent with the focus on the self is Kohut's hypothesis that healthy narcissism has its own lines of continuing development, appearing in both individual and group life. Intrinsic to the group is the development of two basic forms of transference: object-narcissism or the idealizing transference ("my group/leader/etc. is the greatest"); and subject-narcissism, holding constant the concept of perfection of a grandiose self. In the self psychology approach, the emergence of these forms of transference is neither confronted as defensive nor rejected as "unreal." In both, the patient's stance is accepted because this is how the patient sees it! Through this acceptance it is suggested that narcissism, seen as emerging on a developmental line separate from that of object relations, can eventuate in humor, creativity, empathy, and wisdom. The sensitive group therapist will thus not "attempt to push group members away from narcissistic issues to object-love" (Stone and Whitman, 1977, p. 345). This is done despite the difficulties for the group or therapist when, for example, a member who in early life was deprived of an idealized relationship to a parental figure now, as an adult, focuses on the therapist exclusively, ignoring peers, in a desperate search for the lost idealized figure. Early narcissistic deprivation may also show itself in the group member who displays archaic grandiosity by taking on a role familiar to all group leaders, that of monopolizer, disrupter, clown, or critic.

Yet, clinical experience has shown that where empathy reaches out instead of criticism, a cohesive self will finally emerge. In the empathic context of trying to understand the other's needs, attempts to capture failed early idealizations will eventuate in the patient's merger with the selfobject's calmness and power, and the mirroring provided by the group and its leader will lead to healthy exhibitionism and heightened self-esteem.

THE PARTICULAR RELEVANCE OF GROUP SELF
PSYCHOLOGY FOR OLDER ADULTS

Groups for elderly persons living in community settings are a relatively new phenomenon. The first reference to such groups appeared just a little over thirty years ago, in 1950 (Parham, Priddy, McGovern, and Richman, 1982). Where groups were used, it was predominantly in institutional settings catering to adults with severe forms of mental or physical deterioration. These groups focused on the development or enhancement of ADL (Activities of Daily Living) skills, necessary to basic survival, rather than on the acquisition of insight and personality change. More than thirty years after the beginning of any kind of group therapy for the elderly, there is still a dearth of knowledge from outside studies or from any precise attempt to delimit processes and results. What is known from clinical anecdotes is that group works—and little else.

Since self psychology is still in its pioneering stage, it is understandable that there is insufficient research on group self psychology and its effectiveness with older adults. Yet it has been our experience that this approach is most beneficial to the elderly. One reason is that older people have often achieved a comfortable status in life and are less concerned with *what they do* than with *who they are* as people (Weiner, Brok, and Snadowsky, 1987). Group self psychology, with its emphasis on the strengthening of the cohesive self, while also focusing on the interpersonal experiences between group members, would seem to foster this strengthening of later-life identity.

In addition, for those in psychotherapy, lifelong struggle with reality may help soften entrenched character styles. Given their maturity, older patients are often able to take a thoughtful, objective view of themselves and others while accepting human frailties and vanities. In the sharing of experiences intrinsic to aging, the process of "partialized mourning" is supported by the therapist and peers as archaic grandiosity—with its need to control all aspects of life and death—is understood and empathically explored (Weiner, 1984). Similarly, with the gradual loss of faculties accepted as natural to aging (the slowing down of reaction time, changes in taste, smell, visual acuity, etc.) a further lack of self-cohesion may be experienced: "I am not my old self anymore." This is literally true, and the injury to self-cohesion may give rise to rage or depression (White, 1984). But where the therapist and the group members offer themselves as reparative selfobjects, it is possible that self-cohesion may be reestablished.

It has been noted that patients who are overly self-preoccupied or unduly exhibitionistic may be more amenable to treatment in later life (Weiner, Brok and Snadowsky, 1987). Group self psychology, with its acceptance of the mirroring, idealizing, and twinship transferences, would appear suited for later-life exhibitionism, needs for admiration, and the encouragement to try new things in a society centered on the young. In the group, the acquisition of "new" self structures is considered possible so that, whereas lifelong selfobject failures have previously been the rule, now, for the first time perhaps, different experiences may be explored. The encouragement of the "twinship" between group member and group member or therapist, the experience of mirroring, the acceptance of the idealization bestowed, and the encouragement of healthy exhibitionism allow for the self to grow among empathic selfobjects much as a marital partner may exist as a critical, much-needed selfobject for the other in a marriage (Schwartzman, 1984b).

Idealization, accepted in self psychology, is considered the positive transference. Where the opposite takes place and the patient mistrusts and feels angry toward the therapist, feels unprotected in the group, and maintains a noncooperative stance, this is considered an empathic failure on the part of the therapist, and a more sensitive tuning in to the patient's real needs is attempted. The therapist realizes that at a critical moment in the patient's experience the patient needs have not been met. The patient needs to feel that his subjective experience is confirmed and validated by a consistently empathic understanding.

Unlike individual therapy, where patients understand that they will be listened to exclusively by the therapist, in group therapy they must establish their presence, carve out their own identity within the group, make themselves known, and assert that their selves exist! Self-failures are empathized with and never criticized; in a self group, the need for empathic selfobjects is recognized, as are the increased dependency needs that accompany aging, even while independence is affirmed. The use of an empathic approach (Kohut, 1982) fostering the building of self-esteem through acceptance of the *patient's* experience of the aging process, is felt to be the most helpful contribution of self psychology. It appears to have immediate and dramatic positive effects upon our patients. That these should be traced over time, as a road for others to follow, is a goal we strive for.

66   *Marcella Bakur Weiner and Marjorie Taggart White*

REFERENCES

Grotjahn, M. (1981), The therapeutic group process in the light of developmental ego psychology. *Group*, 5:11–16.

Harwood, I. H. (1983), The application of self psychology concepts to group psychotherapy. *Internat. J. Group Psychother.*, 33:469–487.

Kohut, H. (1971), *The Analysis of the Self.* New York: International Universities Press.

——— (1982), Introspection, empathy, and the semi-circle of mental health. *Internat. J. Psycho-Anal.*, 63:395–407.

——— (1984), *How Does Analysis Cure?*, ed. A. Goldberg & P. E. Stepansky. Chicago: University of Chicago Press.

Parham, I. A., Priddy, J. M., McGovern, T. V., & Richman, C. M. (1982), Group psychotherapy with the elderly: Problems and prospects. *Psychotherapy: Theory, Research & Practice*, 19:437–443.

Schwartzman, G. (1984a), The use of the group as self-object. *Internat. J. Group Psychother.*, 34:229–241.

——— (1984b), Narcissistic transferences: Implications for the treatment of couples. *Dynamic Psychother.*, 2:5–14.

Stone, W. N., & Whitman, R. M. (1977), Contributions to the psychology of the self to group process and group therapy. *Internat. J. Group Psychother.*, 27:343–359.

Weiner, M. B. (1984), Aging as ongoing adaptation to partial loss. In: *The Life-Threatened Elderly*, ed. M. Tallmer. New York: Columbia University Press, pp. 31–39.

——— Brok, A. J., & Snadowsky, A. M. (1987), *Working with the Aged*, rev. ed. New York: Prentice-Hall.

White, M. T. (1984), Discussion of: Narcisstic transferences: Implications for the treatment of couples, by Gertrude Schwartzman. *Dynamic Psychother.*, 2:15–17.

——— Weiner, M. B. (1986), *The Theory and Practice of Self Psychology.* New York: Brunner/Mazel.

5

Psychodynamic Group Therapy with the Active Elderly: A Preliminary Investigation

LESLIE M. LOTHSTEIN, Ph.D.

Karl Abraham's 1919 paper, "The Applicability of Psycho-analytic Treatment to Patients at an Advanced Age," took issue with a central tenet of Freudian psychoanalysis: that in the aged "mental processes were too rigidly established for favorable treatment results" (Kahana, 1979, p. 72). Indeed, Freud had been reluctant to treat persons over forty-five using classical technique or even to employ a psychodynamically oriented psychotherapy with this age group. Fortunately, Abraham's ideas were well received and inspired others to conduct psychoanalytic and psychodynamic psychotherapy with the aged (Jelliffe, 1925; Wayne, 1953; Goldfarb, 1955; Grotjahn, 1955; Meerloo, 1955b; Segal, 1958; Berezin and Cath, 1965; Berezin, 1972; Hiatt, 1972; King, 1974; Sandler, 1978; Blum and Tross, 1980; Goodstein, 1982).

Indeed, by the 1970s the fields of geriatric psychiatry and gerontology were well defined and the issue of whether certain elderly patients could benefit from a psychodynamic therapy was moot (Pfeiffer, 1971; Lawton, 1976; Zinberg and Kaufman, 1978; Poon, 1980). However, to successfully employ a psychodynamic therapy with an aged patient the therapist must select appropriate patients and be aware of how certain life cycle themes affect the elderly's treatment (Berezin and Cath, 1965) and, more specifically, their transference reactions (King, 1980).

In the majority of psychotherapy cases reported in the literature the patients were treated in individual psychotherapy. Given the effects of social isolation, disengagement, and depletion on the aged

(Lazarus, 1980), the transformations of narcissism in the elderly (Busse, 1975; Bressler-Feiner, 1981), changes in body image, the major conflicts of the aged centering on generativity vs. self-absorption and integrity vs. despair (Erikson, 1963), and increased dependency issues, one would have thought that psychodynamically oriented group therapy would have played a more significant role in the psychotherapeutic treatment of older persons. However, while group psychotherapy with the elderly has been employed for over thirty years (Parham, Priddy, McGovern, and Richman, 1982), the focus has been almost entirely on supportive techniques (Cooper, 1984), institutional group treatment (Wolff, 1961; Burnside, 1971, 1978), and the treatment of the psychotically disturbed (Silver, 1950; Yalom and Terrazas, 1968) or neurologically impaired (Meerloo, 1955a). A number of group therapy studies have focused also on the treatment of diverse groups of elderly outpatients (Linden, 1955; Liederman and Green, 1965; Berger and Berger, 1972; Goldfarb, 1972). While some group work has even been done with the well elderly (Lieberman and Gourash, 1979), the focus has been primarily on treating the very ill or frail elderly.

In this paper I will describe a project carried out at University Hospitals of Cleveland (Case Western Reserve University, Department of Psychiatry) to reach out to the active elderly who would not have found their way into a traditional psychiatric outpatient service, and to provide them with a psychodynamically oriented group therapy experience. The active elderly are defined as that group of patients over sixty years of age who may have serious physical or emotional illness but are not incapacitated by it. These individuals lead fully independent lives, are retired or near retirement, are autonomous individuals, and have an expressed wish to learn more about themselves interpersonally so that they may lead fuller and more satisfying lives. It is hoped that this paper will shed light on the importance of providing a psychodynamically oriented group therapy approach to a select number of active elderly individuals.

THE PROJECT

During 1981 our Psychiatry Outpatient clinic recorded 907 new visits, of which 99 were from patients over the age of sixty. These visits accounted for only 10 percent of the total number of outpatients seen. Moreover, the vast majority of these older patients were diagnosed as cognitively disturbed. Typically, these patients were referred for neuropsychological assessment, psychiatric assessment of psychotic functioning, or evaluation for placement in a nursing care facility. While some patients were placed on medication for their psychiatric symptoms, only a handful were treated in psychotherapy (none were seen intensively). Typically, older patients who were referred for psychotherapy were seen supportively and for a limited time (in contrast to younger patients, who were seen in intensive psychodynamically oriented therapy). In order to reach out to active elderly patients who might benefit from a psychodynamically oriented psychotherapy, an advertisement was placed in several newspapers describing the formation of a group therapy treatment program for people over sixty who were leading active lives but were experiencing feelings of loneliness and isolation, and problems with social relationships. Fees were set on a sliding scale.

Thirty-nine individuals responded to this advertisement (thirty-one women and eight men). Eventually, seven women and four men were accepted into the program (28 percent of those who responded). Criteria for exclusion included: (1) dementia or gross neurological impairment; (2) emotional pathology that would severely compromise interpersonal interaction (e.g., psychosis or schizophrenia); (3) incapacitating depression or profound character pathology that would preclude successful group interaction.

The twenty-eight who did not participate in the program were a rather diverse group. Two were referred for further evaluation of sensory and neurological disorders, four for sex therapy, seven for individual or couples therapy, and three for drug therapy. Eleven were in fact accepted but dropped out after the initial interview. Only one respondent was judged acutely psychotic and in need of hospitalization, which he refused. One caller (not included in the statistics) thought we were hiring the aged, having mistakenly read "sliding fee scale" as an employment opportunity.

The 28 percent initial dropout rate (eleven respondents) is within the expected range of group therapy dropouts during the referral process (Lothstein, 1978). It was our impression that many of these potential group therapy patients benefited from their limited contact with the clinic. For example, in the one session she attended, a woman in her late seventies told of a profound early childhood loss that left her feeling depressed and isolated even today. She told of witnessing her family murdered in Russia and how she had been raised in a succession of orphanages. Currently she lived alone in an apartment; this was her first real contact since her husband's death a few years previous. While she decided it would be too painful to engage other fellow sufferers in group therapy, she valued her brief contact with the evaluator. As reported, only one patient, a male in his sixties, was actively psychotic and needed to be seen on an emergency basis. In effect, the advertisement had provided us a spectrum of patients who were homogeneous with respect to age and heterogeneous with respect to all other variables (with the exception of race, in that only one black person, a woman, responded to the advertisement).

Two short-term psychodynamically oriented groups (of five months' duration) were organized. The groups met weekly for an hour and a half. Group I consisted of four patients (three women and one man) whose average age was sixty-eight, while Group II consisted of seven patients (four women and three men) whose average age was sixty-nine. Both were coled by psychologists (three interns and a staff psychologist). The focus of the groups was on symptom relief and improved interpersonal functioning through insight and understanding. At termination, several of the patients expressed a desire to continue in group therapy. Consequently, a single long-term group was formed involving male and female cotherapists (one leader from each of the two groups). In addition, another female intern was included as a leader. It is this group, now in its third year, that is the focus of this chapter.

THE GROUP

The therapy group comprises seven individuals (three men and four women). The average age is sixty-six (range: fifty-seven to seventy-two). The youngest patient (age fifty-five at the time of entry into the group) had lied about his age because he so desperately wanted a group therapy approach to his problems. The group consists of six whites and one black (a woman). They range in education from high school through graduate school and have engaged in a variety of professions, from librarian to lawyer. Table 5.1 summarizes the demography of the group.

THE PATIENTS

Phyllis, a seventy-two-year-old spinster, lives alone with her pet rabbits. Up until two years ago she nurtured her mother in a symbiotic

TABLE 5.1

Demographic Characteristics of Group Therapy Patients

Name	Age	Race	Education	Diagnosis	Prior Treatment	Medication	Medical Illnesses	Occupation	Object Relationships
Phyllis	72	W	B.A.	Dysthymic disorder	Individual and hypnosis	antihypertensive	cataracts overweight	Librarian/ Author	F: seduced/abandoned M: symbiotic
Richard	62	W	B.A., M.S.	Dysthymic disorder	Gestalt Sensitivity Counseling	antihypertensive cardiac	high BP heart condition	Engineer	F: abandoned age 6–11 M: died when he was 6 in childbirth
Barbara	71	W	High-Sch	Atypical depression	Psychiatric hospitalization Counseling	antidepressants numerous medicines for chronic illnesses	chronic illnesses (congenitally absent thyroid, breast cancer, hip replacement, detached retina, etc.)	Office manager	F: suicided, pt. 13 M: suicided, pt. 15
Toni	64	B	High-Sch	Agoraphobia Obs-comp	Behavior therapy Counseling	antidepressants	chronic anxiety	Stenographer	F: ambivalent M: ambivalent
Faye	67	W	High-Sch	Dysthymic disorder	None	antihypertensive Tagamet	high BP ulcers	Housewife	F: warm/supportive M: warm/supportive
Frank	69	W	High-Sch	Somatization disorder Passive-dependent	Self-help groups Relaxation and Behavioral Rx	antihypertensive cardiac medicines (over medicated)	chronic ailments heart condition arthritis	Detective	F: mean/hateful M: absent
Harry	57	W	B.A., L.L.B.	Borderline personality	Many supportive therapies	antihypertensive medicines for intestinal ailments	high BP gastrointestinal	Attorney	F: "little Hitler" M: overindulging

relationship. Her mother's death left Phyllis depressed, suicidal, alone, and fragmented. A librarian by profession, Phyllis is the group aesthete. She identifies as a creative but lost soul. In the group she reads poetry aloud and quotes literary sources. She had hoped that group therapy might help her feel whole again and temper her anger and bitterness. However, upon entering the group she turned people off by interrupting conversations and brushing people off. The group reacts to Phyllis as a fragile, almost brittle person. When not engaged in poetic reveries, morbid discussions, or tearful episodes, Phyllis idolized Harry, Richard, and myself and praised and supported Harry in a compulsive way. She told the group that the last time she felt any stirrings of lust was over forty years ago, and that as far as love was concerned she had died a long time ago. The group saw her as a martyr, the group mother, and the poet.

Harry, a fifty-seven-year-old attorney, is the group comedian. It was he who lied about his age in order to become a group member; he felt that his primary difficulties were with social relationships. Charming, witty, yet extremely masochistic, Harry is chronically anxious, phobic, and depressed. Unable to describe how he feels, Harry either retreats to a hypomanic defense and charms the group with his humor or goes into lengthy monologues about what a poor soul he is. He sees his masculinity as defective and feels inadequate and insecure in all of his relationships. Unable to assert himself at home or at work, he feels profoundly humiliated and depressed. He described his youth as one of torment and terror. He viewed his father as a nazi who brutalized the family. Consequently, as a teenager he feared his sexual and aggressive impulses and lived in horror of nuclear war. His high level of anxiety, panic, fright, and terror (combined with inadequate social relationships) suggested a borderline organization of his object relations. In the group he competes with Richard, feels inadequate toward Frank, is infatuated with Phyllis, and tries to rescue Toni.

Faye, a sixty-seven-year-old woman, was referred for group therapy by her sister, who told her that she distorted other people's comments about her and needed to straighten out her "sick" thoughts that no one cared for her. A profoundly loyal, devoted, almost slavish wife and mother, Faye was also an extremely jealous, bitter, and envious woman. Faye felt estranged and isolated from her "one and only son" and excluded by her daughter-in-law (when in fact there is clear evidence that this was not the case). She viewed herself as a helpless individual who was unassertive and easily hurt. Now that her husband was partially retired, she found herself resenting him and preoccupied with all the wrongs in their marriage (especially the fact that he self-ishly controlled her sexually and deprived her of sexual fulfillment). Upon entering the group she gave advice to everyone. In the course of the group Faye developed an idealizing relationship toward Richard and myself, cared for Phyllis and Toni, and avoided Frank and Barbara. She alternated between impatience and caring, espousing a tough attitude toward love while concealing a deep and hurtful feeling of being unloved.

Richard, a retired engineer, was the leader of the group. An intelligent, assertive, though compulsively fumbling man who was often preoccupied, he was initially adored and idolized by the group. Having experienced the fruits of Gestalt therapy and sensitivity training on his job, Richard used his psychological savvy to seduce the others so that he could lead the group. Richard reported that his recent difficulties had begun after his retirement, when his wife started working; he had fallen apart, fearing he was fragmenting and going crazy. An overzealous individual, he portrayed himself as a lost child in search of its mother. Alternating between helper, facilitator, sage, and seer, Richard was stopped dead in his tracks by therapeutic interpretations that focused on his need to re-create a childhood scenario in which he was constantly searching for his dead mother (who had died in childbirth when he was six years old). He adored the women in the group (with the exception of Phyllis) and often asked them out to lunch; cared for and supported Frank; evolved a competitive relationship with Harry; and ignored or belittled Phyllis. He was in love with one of the female therapists and idealized the male therapist.

Toni, the only black patient in the group, was the silent member. An extremely attractive "grandmother," Toni came to each group dressed in tight and flattering clothing and wore four-inch heels (even in winter). An obsessive-compulsive woman, Toni had many phobias. She avoided intimacy with everyone, including her forty-year-old lover. At the start of each session she would fumble through her purse and write notes to herself. When asked a question she would nervously refuse to answer, claiming that her mind had gone blank. She would then feel humiliated and embarrassed. Over the past decade she had raised her only daughter's two children (both girls), who were now "boy crazy" and pregnant. Home life was miserable. The group reacted to Toni by first protecting her and then becoming annoyed by her refusal to fully participate. Toni admired Richard but used her feelings of social inferiority to distance herself from the group. When Barbara entered the group Toni felt she had an ally in that both of them were quiet. However, when Barbara opened up to the group Toni became visibly upset and requested individual treatment to deal with her inhibitions. While the men expressed feelings of attraction to Toni, she pretended not to notice (though she continues to be viewed as a tantalizing, seductive object by the men). Once, when the group was talking about hidden conflicts and wild impulses, Toni became shaken and welts formed over her body. When the interpretation was made that she could allow her feelings to surface and be recognized by others only as physical symptoms (because of the dangers involved in allowing the intensity of her affect to be recognized by herself or others), the welts disappeared.

Frank, who never missed a group session, viewed himself as a "goofball," a nickname his father had given him. He had two homes, one in a poverty-stricken area and the other in the emergency room. Prior to entering the group he was seen at the ER every other day. Although he was diagnosed as having severe vascular problems, high blood pressure, cardiac illness, and "cerebral atrophy," he tended to exaggerate his symptoms and was viewed by physicians as a crank and a complainer. Throughout his life he experienced severe anxiety and panic attacks. In order to escape from his catastrophic feelings of dread, he converted these feelings to somatic symptoms and set off for the ER where he would be cared for. For the first month of group therapy all he talked about was his body, how poor he was, and how awful his wife was. When he finally talked about his personal problems, it was clear that he was a profoundly burdened man with low self-esteem, whose role as a martyr provided him his only modicum of self-respect. At home he nurtured an epileptic son, cared for a depressed daughter, and managed his wife, who was alcoholic and acutely suicidal. He told the group that his aim was to fix everything in the house so that when he died the family wouldn't fall apart (a theme with symbolic meaning for his role in the group). While Frank was very passive-dependent and avoided criticism, he was also a very jealous and envious man who idolized powerful men. In the group he developed a mirror and idealizing transference to Richard and myself and became cognitively disorganized and illogical whenever Richard was away from the group. Phyllis despised him and periodically engaged him in battle.

Barbara, the newest member of the group, had been psychiatrically hospitalized for a severe depression just before entering the group. A chronically ill woman, she had spent a large portion of her life in hospitals. Indeed, hospitals were like a second home to her. She saw herself as an "ugly Dutch brat" (her mother's epithet), a sickly, frail creature who would soon die. Her family life was no less tragic than her medical health. During her adolescence both parents had committed suicide, which left her psychologically numb. Having lost contact with an older sister, she was now alone in the world. In an effort to cope with feelings of despair Barbara wrote poetry and kept a journal. She immersed herself in her office work and dedicated herself to her boss, whose recent winter trip had precipitated her breakdown. In the group she sat stonefaced and rarely initiated conversation. However, when group members encouraged her she engaged them in lively, witty, and enlightened conversation. While she idealized the male members of the group, she was also the most patient and supportive group member (always alleviating the group's guilt). A survivor, she now lived with two other aged adults (a man and woman) in a communal arrangement which our group referred to as "Three's Company."

IMPAIRED NARCISSISTIC EQUILIBRIUM: TWINSHIPS AND THE MOTIVE FOR GROUP THERAPY

Each of the patients who entered group therapy had suffered either a recent major loss or a series of losses that served as the motivation for entering therapy. Table 5.2 summarizes the major losses that precipitated the group members' entry into group therapy. While it is not unusual for individuals to seek help when in acute distress secondary to a loss, abandonment, or death, why these active elderly patients chose group therapy was not immediately obvious. However, after analysis of the participants' transferences it became apparent that they had chosen group therapy in order to overcome their sense of isolation, resolve their profound dependency conflicts, and restore their impaired narcissistic equilibrium (Lazarus, 1980; Harwood, 1983).

The following clinical example underscores the importance of group therapy for restoring an active elderly patient's narcissistic balance. At various times in the therapy Frank's verbal behavior suggested the possibility of an incipient senile dementia. He had difficulty

TABLE 5.2

Preciptants for Entering Group Therapy

Name	Precipitant
Phyllis	Death of mother, who was her sole object
Barbara	Emotional withdrawal of her sole object
Toni	Retirement and removal from her social world
Faye	Emotional disengagement of daughter-in-law coupled with husband's retirement
Frank	Disengagement by physician from his case, removal from position of respect at job
Harry	Wife's special relationship with a woman friend, children moving away, sense of emptiness
Richard	Retirement, wife taking job

verbalizing material, was forgetful, illogical, and often produced free associative material which was quite regressive. The therapists noted that he was most vulnerable whenever Richard was away from the group. At one point Richard was away for two three-week periods during which Frank's behavior was so worrisome that we referred him for neuropsychological testing. The results, which were within normal limits, arrived two weeks after Richard had returned to group and Frank's bizarre behavior had stopped. Frank had developed a mirror and idealizing transference to Richard and his image of Richard provided him an inner sense of self-cohesion. When Richard went away, Frank's object constancy failed (a phenomenon which was selectively focused on Richard as Frank's object constancy was not impaired in other situations). Subsequently, Frank's thinking fragmented (which was exactly what Richard experienced when his wife went to work and he feared he was going crazy). The Richard-Frank relationship represented a twinship or merger (Kohut and Wolff, 1978) in which selfobject transferences were evident (involving parataxic distortions and regressive material in which both parties reenacted their precipitating crises through the other). By projecting his central conflict of abandonment anxiety onto Frank (through the defense mechanism of projective identification), Richard was able to separate from the group and to travel in safety. An interpretation of the Richard-Frank twinship allowed them both to restore their narcissistic equilibrium. The group was then better able to understand how losses and changes in relationships led to feelings of fragmentation, isolation, self-absorption, and despair (by lowering one's self-esteem and self-worth and impairing one's narcissistic equilibrium).

Another clinical example, focusing on the restoration of narcissistic equilibrium through falling and being in love, underscores the importance of group therapy in mobilizing and consolidating self-cohesion around such narcissistic issues as being admired, appreciated, needed, idealized, and loved. In effect, the patient's narcissistic balance is restored, and a vital self created, through the group's recognition, and support, of each individual's need to have aspects of their grandiose-exhibitionistic self confirmed.

Phyllis announced to the group that since her mother died she felt empty and alone. She felt as if she had lost her only friend. While she was aware that her lifelong tie with her mother was "strange," it was the focus of her life. Indeed, she had not dated in forty years and viewed herself as a wilted flower who would never love again. As she involved herself with other members of the group she began to refer to the "group" as a "family" which could "replace" her mother, thereby allowing her to gratify her need for symbiotic union while maintaining her self-cohesion. Without this symbiotic tie she felt depressed, empty, worthless, and dead. When she was most distressed she read the group a poem. Afterward she felt alive, vital, and understood. Harry, who admired Phyllis, told her she was beautiful, intelligent, and lovable (something no man had ever told her). At one point he even told her, "If I were single I would marry you." Like Phyllis, he wrote poems. In the group he verbalized his admiration and respect for her, mirroring her self system and providing gratification of her grandiose-exhibitionistic needs. In turn she praised Harry and protected him from any group criticism (thereby repairing his image of mother who left him unprotected in the face of father's tirades). A mutual mirroring and idealizing transference ensued which excluded other group members. Harry told the group how his wife, like his mother, was never able to understand and empathize with him. Only Phyllis was capable of understanding him. He told the group of his marital frustrations. Once he stayed up all night filled with anxiety. In the morning his wife commented on how well he looked and ignored his pleas that she recognize his real emotional needs. When he became despairing and morose his wife would feed him a special cookie, a morsel which tempted him but left him more enraged. When his wife began a doting relationship with another woman he found himself rageful and impotent. The Phyllis-Harry twinship provided each of them an opportunity to repair the damages to their overburdened self systems and feel vital and loved. At one point Phyllis announced to the group that she had actually fallen in love with someone outside the group. Her relationship with Harry had bolstered her self-esteem and led to the emergence of a vital, nondepressed self system which was capable of falling in love.

While subgrouping is traditionally seen as impairing group cohesiveness the effect in this group was quite different. Indeed, what stood out was the reparative effects such pairings, or twinships, had in restoring the individual's narcissistic equilibrium. While some group members commented on the exclusiveness of the pairings (and expressed a variety of feelings ranging from jealousy and envy to genuine support) they respected the way in which the subgrouping led to a more cohesive and vital self system. Given the fact that some of the major developmental conflicts of the elderly focus on Erikson's (1963) bipolar variables (generativity vs. self absorption and integrity vs. despair) one can appreciate the object-relations dilemmas of the elderly. That is, the self system must be maintained and elaborated via the establishment of mutually satisfying object ties just at a time in the life cycle when such object ties are being broken. In this sense, the elderly are particularly vulnerable to being overwhelmed by feelings of self fragmentation. Not only may they find themselves succumbing to self-absorption and despair secondary to constant shifts in their object ties, but their increased dependency further lowers their self-esteem and sense of autonomy (issues which are then reflected in shifts in their narcissistic equilibrium). Group therapy, by providing a source of objects, and the possibility of developing rewarding object ties, allows the active elderly to reintegrate their self systems and overcome their sense of isolation and despair.

CAN THERE BE FAVORABLE TREATMENT RESULTS WITH THE AGED?

Kahana (1980), quoted Freud as saying that in the aged "mental processes were too rigidly established for favorable treatment results." Is this a tenable hypothesis? Consider the following clinical material.

Richard entered group fearing he "was going crazy and frag-menting" when his wife, after his retirement, went to work. While he intellectually knew that it was all right for his wife to work he was emotionally distraught and frantic. In the course of his group therapy the following story emerged. When Richard was six his mother gave birth to his sister. The whole extended family celebrated the event joyously. The next day a somber mood prevailed. The family was distraught. Richard was whisked away from his family and for the next five years lived in foster homes. Apparently, his mother had developed an embolism, one day postpartum, and died. His father, unable to cope with the loss, gave up Richard and his sister to two separate families to raise. When Richard was eleven his father showed up with two women and asked him which one he wanted to be his mother. Of course he couldn't choose. But the family was reunited. In the course of his life Richard was constantly searching for his dead mother. He married a woman who looked like her and, throughout his adult life, became infatuated with, and involved with women who looked like mother.

In the course of his treatment it became apparent that his en-actment of this search left people confused and annoyed with him. His actions were perceived as ungenuine and his motivations were suspect. Repeated interpretations enabled Richard to stop acting out and to bear the pain and anguish of his past. Once he told the group about an impending family reunion, which his daughter, her husband and child were driving a long distance to attend. He was frantic and panicked that they would die, though he was aware of the irrationality of this idea. When the interpretation was made that the family's com-ing together for a celebration brought up old memories from when he was six of how a festive occasion could turn into a tragedy Richard broke down and wept. Repeated interpretations not only freed him from this core conflict but also led to changes in other aspects of his self and ego functioning. He became less compulsive and controlling; less self absorbed and egocentric; gave up acting out his core neurotic fantasy of reunion with mother; and began to listen carefully to what others said.

AGING AND THE THIRD PHASE OF SEPARATION-INDIVIDUATION

Many of the group patients were actively struggling with ambiv-alent feelings related to their increased dependency status. One patient in Group I, Brenda, who died just after the group terminated, was fiercely struggling with her new dependency status. She was a creative, intelligent, resourceful woman who had always been independent. During her life she had traveled alone to Europe and managed a successful career. Now that she had leukemia she was too weak to even drive her own car. In group she shook her fists and fought with the men; while at home she attempted to cope with her dependency fears by engaging her husband in knockdown fights. Although she died just after the group terminated, we learned that she was fighting both her illness and her dependency needs right to the end. Another patient from Group II, Howard, was a loyal and obedient son. He made daily trips to the nursing home to provide basic care for his ninety-year-old mother. His regressive experience with mother (including having to fecally disempact her) fostered an intolerable symbiotic union which left him feeling as if he had no separate existence. For other patients, retirement and/or physical illness (Richard, Frank, Barbara), sensory impairment (Phyllis, Barbara), or emotional stress and environmental factors (Harry and Faye) had led to increased dependency feelings which were intolerable.

Some of our patients reported that their grown children acted as if they were the parents; reversing the traditional roles and usurping their parents' autonomy (even before they really needed help from their children). Others found themselves having an aged parent move in with them (or being preoccupied with them psychologically). Now in their sixties their parents (in the eighties and nineties) treated them as children; demanding to know where they were going and when they would be back. As a consequence of their newly discovered dependency many of the elderly were also asked to relinquish autonomous functioning which was necessary for the maintenance of their self-esteem. In effect, there was very little outlet for their anger and guilt over their new dependency status.

In this phase of psychosocial development the aged are asked to once again struggle with separation-individuation issues, but from a different perspective. Now the issue becomes one of accepting their newfound dependency status without having to lose their separate identity. Their guilt over giving in to their dependency needs often became a focus of the group process. Feelings of depression, rage, ambivalence, and guilt which were previously associated with stage I (Mahler, 1972) and stage II (Blos, 1979) separation-individuation processes are still evident for the elderly in stage III but the process is reversed, with attachment and dependency, not separation, being the goal. The paradox of this stage is that throughout the life cycle individuals are asked to individuate, be ambitious, self-interested, successful, and separate. Now the individual is asked to relinquish those goals and allow oneself to merge with a caretaker while also maintaining a sense of self-identity. The only precedent for this life cycle task is in infancy with the maternal bond. Group therapists must be aware of the dangers involved in resolving this potentially regressive developmental task, that is, having to cope with the need to yield and passively surrender to caretakers and the conflicts and pressures it places on each group member. It appears from our experience that group therapy, in contrast to individual therapy, may allow a person's dependency needs to unfold in a safe and caring environment. In individual therapy the person's guilt over dependency needs may lead to either intense depressive states (over loss of self-esteem and autonomy) or excessive dependence on the therapist (which can be antitherapeutic). In group therapy issues of self-identity and self-worth are encouraged to develop in the context of the welcomed dependency relationships among group members. The group lessens the individuals' superego burdens and thereby lessens their guilt associated with the completion of this life cycle task. One of the responsibilities of the group therapist is to provide the appropriate interpretations to the group so that the dependency issues can flourish alongside the individuation issues (thereby allowing the aging patient to view this stage as a new challenge to the growth of the self system throughout the life cycle rather than as evidence that the self is either depleted or dead).

GROUP PROCESS ISSUES

From the very outset of the groups the patients showed a concern and caring for each other. Issues of competitiveness, rivalry, and aggression, which are generally present in beginning groups of young adults, were absent in these groups. While there is the possibility that this was due to subtle countertransference issues it is unlikely. Rather, it was the impression of all leaders that the tasks of our elderly patients were different. All of them had an expressed desire to seek out and have the capacity for object relationships which were meaningful and sustaining. As the group progressed into its second year aggressive and competitive issues did emerge. Indeed, these issues became a central focus of the group's work. It is our impression that one ought not to treat the elderly's altruistic motives (at the beginning of group therapy) as purely defensive. While such behaviors certainly facilitated the development of a therapeutic alliance they also were socially adaptive (perhaps developmentally necessary) in order to link them with important objects.

By the beginning of the second year issues of competition and aggression did emerge; with the focus typically centering on feelings of disappointment about their children. These were also viewed as transference issues and interpreted in terms of rivalry and envy of the younger therapists (who were viewed as having a whole life in front of them). The youthfulness of the female therapists also caused many of the female patients to feel envious. Group members projected erotic and aggressive (assertive) feelings onto the female therapists and envied their status. There was open talk about what wonderful and exciting careers and sexual lives the female therapists had. When the male members of the group flirted with the female therapists but not with the women patients this naturally led to feelings of jealousy.

LEADERSHIP ISSUES

Group therapists must modify some of their tactics and techniques with this age group. Typically the leaders are considerably younger than the patients. While the age differences between the leaders and patients necessitates the recognition of how certain unique transference and countertransference issues emerge, those age differences are not insurmountable. In our three groups the age differences were less a factor than the gender differences. Although the female therapists were about thirty-five years younger than their patients and the male therapist twenty-five years younger, the critical factor was gender. The patients tended to refer to the male leader as doctor and the female leaders as "girls," an epithet that aroused considerable anger among the female coleaders and led to splitting in the leadership. Typically, the group members devalued what the women leaders had to offer, though in the course of any one group they may have asked the female leaders' opinions and feedback and acknowledged that they benefited from their interpretations. The gender gap theme was highlighted by the groups' habit of calling only the female leaders by their first names. While an analysis of this group behavior led to the groups' acknowledging the role status of the female leaders as "doctors too," they never fully accepted the women as true leaders. For example, Frank called the male leader by his title, doctor, a symbolic name which facilitated Frank's idealizing transference to a powerful male figure (which allowed him to feel whole and intact while also distancing him from his feelings). Frank's ambivalence toward women emerged in his calling the female leaders "girls," treating them as sex objects, and even sarcastically belittling one of them. Eventually, he acknowledged their "doctor" status when he realized that there were "three doctors caring for me" (an idea which made him feel exalted). However, he never fully accepted the women as leaders and always asked the male leader questions when he wanted a "real answer." Phyllis regarded the female leaders as "children," not as real doctors and looked to the male leader for understanding and insight (in spite of the fact that she transferred, with her female therapist, from another group into this one). Moreover, Richard claimed that although he had learned a lot from the female leaders "they were only women and couldn't help him. Girls have no power." When the women leaders terminated from the group he was bitter and disappointed. He dealt with their loss by depreciating them, a theme which had personal meaning and was also related to the groups' transference to the mother figure as a powerful, destructive, and nurturing symbol. While there were many aspects of the meaning of the group's relationship to the female leaders, one could not help but wonder how this related to the issue of increased dependency: that is, the group's need to fend off the mother figure (which symbolically represented their increased dependency status) thereby preserving their sense of self-identity. In one of the earlier groups this conflict was acted out by the male patients' attempts to force the women patients to leave the group. Once this was interpreted as an acting out of the group members' feared increased dependency, the need to forcefully expel the women stopped. Another male group member acted out this theme in relation to his wife and transferred onto the female therapists. He related how his wife scolded him for wetting the toilet seat when he peed. Because he feared her aggression and rejection, he compromised by sitting to urinate. While this behavior might have previously threatened his male identity this was no longer the case. Indeed, he was now relieved of the anxiety that she might leave him.

Group therapists must be active and directive with their elderly patients. They must also be careful not to assume control of their patient's ego functions. While silent, distant leadership runs the risk of losing the group through a high dropout rate, a too active leadership will infantilize the group (making it pathologically dependent on the leader) and will lead to a supportive rather than a dynamic group therapy.

CHANGES IN PATIENT FUNCTIONING: NEW BEGINNINGS

Throughout the course of the group, members asked the leaders for guidance and advice to solve their life problems. They seemed to be looking to the leaders as surrogate parents to provide a magical "truth serum" (as Phyllis put it) to cure them. The fact that many of them were parents (71 percent) and in the advice-giving business, were well versed in the self-help literature, and listened to the psychological jockeys on the radio (who told them exactly what to do with their lives) provided them a leadership model in which omnipotence, grandiosity, and charisma were stressed. Had we given into the group's demands for advice and guidance, we might have prematurely reinforced certain dependency issues and provided them a negative model of change based on infantile dependence and omnipotent leadership.

While no single factor accounted for the variety of changes in patient functioning, it appeared that the necessary condition for change involved the formation of a positive group climate and atmosphere which facilitated group cohesiveness. This group climate, often referred to by our patients as a "new family" (which was accepting and nonjudgmental, thereby lessening group guilt), formed a type of holding environment which allowed group members to experiment with new ideas and behaviors and give up old defenses. In retrospect, it appeared that a time-limited group experience (the two five-month groups) did not allow the sense of being a "family" to develop. There was simply not enough time. Group therapists should take this into account when organizing group therapy for the active elderly.

Some of the changes that took place in the patients included the following:

Phyllis stopped intellectualizing and became more feeling oriented; improved her peer relations; was less bitter and vengeful; resolved her guilt over the symbiotic relationship with her mother; became less of a martyr and learned to take of herself; and fell in love.

Richard controlled his acting out; confronted, and mostly resolved, his neurotic transference as a "motherless child" in search of a mother imago; gained self-cohesion; was better able to tolerate losses and separations; confronted his need to control and dominate others (stopped monopolizing the group with vague and confusing intellectualizations); and was able to contact relatives and renew family ties.

Frank made significantly fewer visits to the emergency room; stopped viewing himself as a complex of bodily symptoms and was able to focus on himself as a person; developed some meaningful object relationships; was more reality oriented vis-à-vis his alcoholic wife; and had more self-esteem.

Harry was less rageful and anxious; was able to focus on feelings; developed a more satisfying relationship with his wife; was less envious and jealous; was able to be more assertive with employees; was less phobic; was able to accept ambivalent feelings and not polarize his feelings; and developed a more realistic self-image.

Faye was able to be more assertive with her husband; feels less depressed and hopeless about the future; has a lessened need for advice and support and is now asking for feedback about the way others experience her; and is less rigid and inflexible in problem solving.

Toni, while making only modest gains, is now able to talk to the group for extended periods of time; attends almost every group session; is more assertive at home with her grandchildren (whom she raises); and states that the group has helped her face up to the problems more realistically. However, she is still overcontrolled and lacks spontaneity, is constricted and overburdened by the group, and anxiously protects herself from responding to group questions.

Barbara, the newest member, has shown the fewest gains. However, she is less confused and depressed and is more spontaneous and open with the group.

Clearly the group therapy experience has been quite successful in helping a variety of active elderly patients resolve their problems in living. While all of the group members feel that they have a lot more to learn about themselves, their gains in psychodynamically oriented group therapy are impressive. Eisdorfer, (1984) reviewing "stereotypes of aging," claims "that older persons are not simply concerned with issues of loss and death, but that they can continue to maintain a rich and vibrant inner life." Our group therapy experience confirms this notion and suggests that not only can they maintain "a rich and vibrant inner life," but that they can augment and change that inner life as well.

REFERENCES

Abraham, K. (1919), The applicability of psycho-analytic treatment to patients at an advanced age. In: *Selected Papers.* New York: Basic Books, 1953, pp. 312–317.
Berezin, M. (1972), Psychodynamic considerations of aging and the aged: An overview. *Amer. J. Psychiat.,* 128:1483–1491.
—— Cath, S., Eds. (1965), *Geriatric Psychiatry: Grief, Loss, and Emotional Disorders in the Aging Process.* New York: International Universities Press.
Berger, M. M., & Berger, L. F. (1972), Psychogeriatric group approaches. In: *Progress in Group and Family Therapy,* ed. C. Sager & H. S. Kaplan. New York: Brunner/Mazel, pp. 737–746.
Blos, P. (1979), *The Adolescent Passage.* New York: International Universities Press.
Blum, J. & Tross, S. (1980), Psychodynamic treatment of the elderly: A review of issues in theory and practice. In: *Annual Review of Gerontology and Geriatrics,* ed. C. Eisdorfer. New York: Springer.
Bressler-Feiner, M. (1981), Narcissism and role loss in older adults. *J. Geriatric Psychiat.,* 14:91–110.
Burnside, I. M. (1971), Long-term group work with the hospitalized aged. *Gerontologist,* 11:213–218.
—— (1978), *Working with the Elderly: Group Processes and Techniques.* North Scituate, Mass.: Duxbury Press.
Busse, E. (1975), Social changes, economic status and the problems of aging. In: *American Handbook of Psychiatry: Vol. VI,* ed. S. Arieti. New York: Basic Books, pp. 947–959.
Cooper, D. (1984), Group psychotherapy with the elderly: Dealing with loss and death. *Amer. J. Psychother.,* 38:203–214.
Eisdorfer, C. (1984), Models of mental health care for the elderly. In: *Geriatric Mental Health,* ed. Abrahams & Crook. Grune & Stratton, pp. 217–227.
Erikson, E. (1963), *Childhood and Society,* rev. ed. New York: Norton.
Goldfarb, A. I. (1955), One aspect of the psychodynamics of the therapeutic situation with aged patients. *Psychoanal. Rev.,* 42:180–187.
—— (1972), Group therapy with the old and the aged. In: *Group Treatment of Mental Illness,* ed. H. I. Kaplan & B. J. Sadock. New York: Dutton, pp. 113–131.
Goodstein, R. (1982), Individual psychotherapy and the elderly. *Psychotherapy: Theory, Research & Practice,* 19:412–418.
Grotjahn, M. (1955), Analytic psychotherapy with the elderly. *Psychoanal. Rev.,* 42:419–427.
Harwood, I. H. (1983), The application of self psychology concepts to group psychotherapy. *Internat. J. Group Psychother.,* 33:469–487.
Hiatt, H. (1972), Dynamic psychotherapy of the aged. *Curr. Psychiatric Therapies,* 12:224–229.
Jelliffe, S. E. (1925), Old age factors in psychoanalytic therapy. *Med. J. Rev.,* 121:7–12.
Kahana, R. (1979), Strategies of dynamic psychotherapy with the wide range of older individuals. *J. Geriatric Psychiat.,* 12:71–100.

King, P. (1974), Notes on the psychoanalysis of older patients: Reappraisal of the potentialities for change during the second half of life. *J. Analyt. Psychol.*, 19:22–37.

—— (1980), The life cycle as indicated by the nature of the transference in the psychoanalysis of the middle-aged and elderly. *Internat. J. Psycho-Anal.*, 61:153–160.

Kohut, H., and Wolf, E. (1978), The disorders of the self and their treatment: An outline. *Internat. J. Psycho-Anal.*, 59:413–425.

Lawton, M. P. (1976), Geropsychological knowledge as a background for psychotherapy with older people, *J. Geriatric Psychiat.*, 9:221–234.

Lazarus, L. W. (1980), Self psychology and psychotherapy with the elderly: Theory and practice. *J. Geriatric Psychiat.*, 13:69–88.

Lieberman, M., & Gourash, N. (1979), Evaluating the effects of change groups on the elderly. *Internat. J. Group Psychother.*, 29:283–304.

Liederman, P. C., & Green, R. (1965), Geriatric outpatient group therapy. *Comprehensive Psychiat.*, 6:51–60.

Linden, M. E. (1955), Transference in gerontologic group psychotherapy: IV. Studies in gerontologic human relations. *Internat. J. Group Psychother.*, 5:61–79.

Lothstein, L. (1978), The group psychotherapy dropout phenomenon revisited. *Amer. J. Psychiat.*, 135:1492–1495.

Mahler, M. (1972), On the first three subphases of the separation-individuation process. *Internat. J. Psycho-Anal.*, 53:333–338.

Meerloo, J. (1955a), Psychotherapy with elderly people. *Geriatrics*, 10:583–587.

—— (1955b), Transference and resistance in geriatric psychotherapy. *Psychoanal. Rev.*, 42:72–82.

Miller, N., & Cohler, B. (1984), Psychodynamic research perspectives on development, psychopathology, and treatment in later life. *Psychoanal. Psychol.*, 1:77–82.

Parham, I. A., Priddy, J. M., McGovern, T. V., and Richman, C. M. (1982), Group psychotherapy with the elderly: Problems and prospects. *Psychotherapy: Theory, Research & Practice*, 19:437–443.

Pfeiffer, E. (1971), Psychotherapy with elderly patients. *Postgrad. Med.*, 50:254–258.

Poon, L. W., Ed. (1980), *Aging in the 1980's: Psychological Issues*. Washington, D.C.: American Psychological Association.

Sandler, A. (1978), Problems in the psychoanalysis of an aging narcissistic patient. *J. Geriatric. Psychiat.*, 11:5–36.

Segal, H. (1958), Fear of death: Notes on the analysis of an old man. *Internat. J. Psycho-Anal.*, 29:178–181.

Silver, A. (1950), Group psychotherapy with senile psychotic patients. *Geriatrics*, 5:147–150.

Wayne, G. (1953), Modified psychoanalytic therapy in senescence. *Psychoanal. Rev.*, 40:99–116.

Wolff, K. (1961), Group psychotherapy with geriatric patients in a Veterans Administration hospital. *Group Psychother.*, 14:85–89.

Yalom, I., & Terrazas, F. (1968), Group therapy for psychotic elderly patients. *Amer. J. Nursing*, 68:1690–1694.

Zinberg, N., and Kaufman, I., Eds. (1978), *Normal Psychology of the Aging Process*, rev. ed. New York: International Universities Press.

6

Growing Old and Growing: Psychodrama with the Elderly

GILBERT A. SCHLOSS, Ph.D., C.S.W.

This chapter is concerned primarily with discussing and describing ways in which psychodrama has been helpful in working with the elderly. Clinical material has been drawn largely from psychodramatically oriented therapy groups I have conducted at the Institute for Sociotherapy in New York. The elderly treated in the group are neither confined nor institutionalized. They live independently or with their adult children. The issues they raise and the problems they present in their therapy groups are similar to those reported in the current literature.

Recently a combination of factors has led to a reexamination by psychological researchers of issues concerning the elderly and a heightened interest by psychotherapists in working with them (Nissenson, 1984). While these factors include an emerging political voice and economic impact (Aiken, 1982), perhaps the most important is the simple fact that more people are living longer. Between 1960 and 1980, the total number of children in our population below fifteen years of age fell 7 percent, while the number of elderly people rose 54 percent (Preston, 1984).

The elderly, identified conventionally as people sixty-five or older, are the fastest growing segment of our population. They are also in many ways the most difficult group to discuss. As well as having as a group all the diversity of intelligence, temperament, and racial characteristics found in children, adolescents, and younger adults, individually they have a long lifetime of educational, social, and environmental experience. And to make generalizations even more difficult, different people age at different rates, depending on such aspects as genetics and health. A major problem is that as a chronologically identified group, the elderly are the most heterogeneous (Brody, 1973). The setting of sixty-five as the threshold of older adulthood, then, is largely arbitrary.

With all the acknowledged diversity, however, certain general statements can still be made. Whatever the individual rate, aging is a universal process. Becoming elderly usually involves a diminution of activities, opportunities, and alternatives. Often there is a slowing down and narrowing of life and an increase in physical ailments. There is usually a lessening of income, which affects both the quality of life and the possibility of obtaining needed services. There is sometimes the loss of a spouse and of peers. Becoming elderly often involves some withdrawal from work and productive activity. Self-esteem can be threatened when elderly parents, who once provided nurturance and guidance themselves, become dependent on their children for care or economic aid.

As well as health problems and personal losses, the elderly have to contend with social stereotypes. Despite greater public awareness in recent years, many still consider senility an inevitable outcome of aging. While there is some short-term memory and attention loss, senility is more often a manifestation of physical problems or psychological withdrawal than the ordinary experience of most elderly persons. Often a lessening of the ability to perform tasks demanding speed or coordination is taken as a loss of intellectual function. Yet when judgment and experience are the criteria, skill levels do not seem to diminish (Brody, 1979). Still, there is a tendency, even among professionals, to routinely pass off the possibly reversible physical or emotional problems of the elderly as natural and inevitable outcomes of aging.

The elderly, as products of the same society, have themselves been influenced by these prejudices. Often they are caught up in stereotypic notions as to their supposedly limited capacities to perform because of advanced age. Though still capable, many elderly persons consign themselves to a life of fewer possibilities and lower productivity than they might desire. They become convinced that wanting a sexual life, exploring new areas of intellectual interest, or attempting new behaviors are not age-appropriate. They feel they will be subjected to ridicule or will feel foolish. Underlying this attitude is the assumption that old age is a time to keep busy and distracted while fading away toward death.

Little wonder, then, that until fairly recently there was no great degree of professional interest in conducting psychotherapy with the elderly. After all, it was thought, dealing with the emotional and psychological problems of the young or middle-aged opens up the opportunity for heightened productivity and a better life. The elderly might experience emotional and psychological stress when faced with loss of status or loved ones at a time in their lives when they are least equipped to deal with that stress. Still, what can psychotherapy really offer them, people whose life has almost passed? As a result of this attitude, mental health services, when available, were largely custodial, involving institutions, agencies, and nursing homes.

Current attitudes have shown marked change (Nissenson, 1984). Far from stressing the elderly's withdrawal of interest in the outside world, an emphasis that marked many studies in the sixties (Cummings and Dean, 1972), or the theoretical depiction of aging as a stage for giving way and preparing for death (Erikson, 1950), the contemporary literature often characterizes life after sixty-five as a period of continued development and growth (Brody, 1973; Aiken, 1982). Unique possibilities exist for the aging individual to find personal satisfaction and productivity.

Though seldom discussed in the literature (Buchanan, 1981; Altman, 1983), psychodrama and related approaches—sociodrama and role playing—are particularly well-suited group therapy modalities for working with the elderly. Psychodrama is flexible. The form allows for psychological exploration that can move easily through time and space, from fantasy to reality. The combination of spontaneous dialogue and focused action allows for the adaptability to individual differences that a heterogeneous population needs. The dramatization of problems can produce an immediacy which often leads both the protagonist and the other group members to a more heightened emotional involvement than is normally available through description or narration. Yet the action is "staged." A drama is created in the moment, thereby evoking a sense of theater. This gives the protagonist an opportunity to gain a perspective he might not have had at the time of the original action. In sociodrama, group members are able to deal with themes of common interest without focusing on an individual member's specific life experience. Role playing and role training offer opportunities for rehearsing activities and discussing the feelings these activities evoke. Elderly group members can experiment with alternative behaviors and receive supportive feedback concerning which behavior appears most effective.

Psychodramatic process also helps older group members enhance their self-esteem by allowing them to use their own experience in helping others. It offers each group member permission to deal with issues of personal concern that others bring up, and the prospect of pooling information to find productive outlets for their energy —productive energy that might otherwise go to waste (Uhlenberg, 1979).

A TYPICAL GROUP INTERACTION

"I must be crazy, or stupid," she sighed. "Or senile. What am I doing talking about going to college at seventy-one? I'm too old. People would laugh at me." Mary, the protagonist, had just reached the point in her psychodrama where she had revealed to the group her hidden wish to return to school and take a degree, only to be stopped short by her own stereotypic attitudes. Mary had grown up with narrow ideas concerning aging and age-appropriateness that now threatened to become self-fulfilling. Her opportunity for personal development was endangered not by limitations imposed by others, or by her physical and economic circumstances, but by her own identification of old age with atrophy rather than growth.

"The students will laugh at a grandmother sitting in their class," Sam said, following the psychodrama director's cue: Sam was playing the role of Mary's adult son. The director then turned to the group and encouraged them to verbalize highly critical statements concerning Mary's plan. Here they assumed the role of a Greek chorus, representative of the opinion Mary feared. Cries of "You're too old," "Sounds like second childhood," "Silly grandma," came from different group members. One turned to another and in a loud stage whisper said, "Did you hear. . . .?"

When different group members called out, Mary's head at first became bowed, as if she couldn't stand up to the weight of their ridicule. Then the group voices had the desired effect of mobilizing her anger. She turned toward them and shouted, "Shut up! You don't know!" She silenced them. She then spoke passionately about her right to pursue her dream.

Suddenly her voice dropped. She turned to Rita, who was playing the role of Mary's wise and knowing self, and said sadly, "What's the good? I'm being silly. I'm too old. I probably won't even live long enough to finish the degree."

"So?" Rita responded. "What will happen then? God will give you an incomplete?"

Mary smiled. "What could be worse?" She began to laugh. The group joined in good-naturedly. The director stopped the action and moved to the final part of the psychodrama, the sharing. In this phase, Mary, who had emerged from the group to become the protagonist, the person on whom the psychodrama was focused, was reintegrated into the group. This was achieved by having the other group members share directly with Mary their own feelings and personal experiences touched off by the psychodrama.

In this portion group members brought up problems related to aging. Many comments concerned situations involving self-stereotyping. Phil, seventy years old, stuttered and stammered for a while, then was able to mention the sexual difficulties he was having with his wife. He enjoyed sex occasionally and wanted to have an active sex life, but felt foolish at his age. His wife thought there was something the matter with him, he admitted. She kept telling him, "Act your age!" Phil's "confession" led Sarah to admit blushingly that she was fighting guilt feelings and the suspicion that she was perverted. Having recently been widowed from a man she felt affection for but had long ceased having sexual relations with, she now found herself, at sixty-seven, beginning to have sexual fantasies once again. Helen, a seventy-year-old widow, talked about wanting to resume painting, which she had given up many years before while she raised her family. Apologetically, she admitted to feeling tired of being the "good mother" and trying to respond to her adult children's needs before her own. "When do I graduate?" she asked. "When do I allow myself to put first what I'm interested in?" She thanked Mary for helping her get in touch with those feelings. Eventually Phil, Helen, and Sarah, each in good time, became protagonists in their own psychodramas.

THE WARM-UP

The components of psychodrama lend themselves particularly well to work with older adults. The first part of the psychodrama, the warm-up, helps break down awkward barriers of silence and encourages the possibility of interaction among older group members in a nonthreatening, sometimes even playful way. The director might ask different group members where they might be, or what they might be doing, if they could be anywhere doing anything. He might point to an empty chair and ask each to imagine someone—famous, fictional, or from their own lives—sitting in the chair and to begin a dialogue. The director might suggest an age regression, in which various members pick an earlier time in their lives, often between one and ten years old, and describe to each other what life was like then in an immediate, sensually oriented way.

Because of the activity and interactional aspects of the warm-up, its functions help raise the group's emotional level. This is an important part of the psychodrama process, as it sets the stage for the emergence of the protagonist: someone in the group indicates, by emotional tone, behavior, or direct statement, that he or she is ready to work on some personal issue. The group member who becomes the protagonist usually displays a heightened emotional intensity. Yet if the protagonist is too much higher than the others, they will not feel connected to her. The presentation will at that point be too strong for them to identify with. The director must therefore make sure that both the protagonist and the group are sufficiently warmed up for group process to operate effectively. Usually, however, once a protagonist is found the warm-up stops and the action portion of the psychodrama begins.

EMERGENCE OF THE PROTAGONIST AND THE ASSIGNMENT OF ROLES

If the director achieves the right emotional balance, the protagonist's emergence will place that person in the dual situation of exploring a personal problem and acting as representative, if not spokesperson, for the group. This dual position is reinforced by the protagonist's movement into dramatic action rather than descriptive narrative. The issues being dealt with take on a greater sense of immediacy, for both protagonist and group, when experienced dramatically. The protagonist draws the group into greater involvement with the action by choosing different group members to play "significant others" in the psychodrama. The director instructs the protagonist to pick a person for a particular role who is reminiscent in some way, no matter how small, of some significant other. The person chosen doesn't have to be the same age or even sex of the person to be portrayed. The resemblance may be physical, but may reside as well in gesture, attitude, or tone of voice. The protagonist's association increases the possibility of more intense interaction with the group member in the psychodrama.

Yet the group member playing, say, the protagonist's mother is in fact not that person. Nor is the protagonist five years old, though the scene being enacted and feelings evoked may originally have occurred at that age. Since the players and the scenes are dramatic re-creations, not the events themselves, they afford the protagonist a measure of perspective even as they allow a level of intensity unavailable through simple narrative.

Although group members are cast in roles according to the protagonist's association, they do not as a rule know personally the characters they are depicting. The protagonist must therefore train group members on the spot to play the significant others accurately enough to satisfy the protagonist's needs. Group members must be shown how the significant others might act or what they might say in different situations. Group members must pick up a "feel" for their roles to the point where they can proceed satisfactorily "in character." In order to train the group members, the protagonist must reverse roles with the significant others in his life and try to express himself from their various points of view. Sometimes this role reversal helps the protagonist transcend the personal standpoint and gain perspective on how others might have felt in the situation being re-created.

Older group members chosen for ancillary roles in the psychodrama also benefit from being cast. For one thing, they are identified as people from whom the protagonist can accept help. This often gives elderly group members a sense of importance and worth so often threatened by retirement and other limits placed on their social roles. Also, because they must follow the protagonist's instructions in order to play their roles effectively, elderly group members usually experience such training as a nonthreatening opportunity to display their desire and ability to learn something new. Since the dialogue beyond the role training is often produced spontaneously, group members must draw on their past experience as son, father, husband, or daughter, mother, wife, thereby giving value to this experience in the present moment. Yet because they are playing another person, this trying on of another point of view may help them gain perspective on their own lives. Finally, if they are helpful, members may experience enhanced self-esteem from the approval given their performance by the protagonist and the group.

SHARING AS EPILOGUE TO THE DRAMA

The sharing at the end of each psychodrama serves several functions. It helps to reintegrate the protagonist into the group by affording needed emotional support. Group members indicate through their participation that the protagonist is not alone in the issues with which he is struggling. They can understand, empathize, and relate what has been depicted to elements in their own lives. The sharing also benefits group members generally. Stimulated by the action they have observed, group members often begin, in the sharing, a new personal exploration. Feeling relief in having mentioned their own problems, they often open up even more in subsequent sessions. When group members share in another's psychodrama, they are usually coming closer to becoming the protagonist in their own.

The benefits of psychodrama are not experienced only by the protagonist, the auxiliary players, and those who share their feelings verbally at the end. For example, Rachel, a sixty-eight-year-old widow, was placed in a chronologically heterogeneous group. As group members in their thirties, forties, and fifties explored issues of concern to them, Rachel remained silent, even in the sharing portion. Yet to judge from her facial expression during the psychodrama, she was interested, involved, and affected. After the sixth or seventh meeting, a group member turned to her and questioned her silence. Rachel responded, saying she knew it was selfish of her but she was enjoying the feeling of not being expected or obligated to take care of everyone in the group. "For so many years," she said, "I'd been a dutiful daughter, then a wife, a mother, and a grandmother. I automatically expected to be called upon to take responsibility for whatever trouble occurs. Or people will get angry at me." She paused and looked around for reassurance. "But not here. Here no one needs me to be their mother. Regardless of my age, I can just be Rachel."

What followed was a psychodrama in which Rachel looked for her "self" in the different supportive roles she played during her life. She found a curious, interested, even flirtatious woman who displayed a lively sense of fun. She explored ways in which these sides of herself could be expressed and enjoyed without being subordinated to other people's needs. In the process she became a more valued and valuable group member.

RETROSPECTION AND UNFINISHED BUSINESS

For the elderly especially, a psychodrama that allows for retrospection is of great use. When a life is reviewed in a relatively short time span, major patterns and themes can be brought to greater awareness. As old wounds, arguments, and conflicts become articulated psychodramatically, they can be placed in a broader context, often allowing the protagonist to reach some sense of closure. Poor choices, accidents, and failures that had rankled in the past lose their significance now or can be seen sometimes as blessings in disguise. When, as with the elderly, the present contains stressful unknowns, the past as reexperienced psychodramatically can bring the protagonist some sense of order.

Harry's age had caught him by surprise. "Suddenly," he admitted to nodding group members, "I was seventy-two years old. And I didn't really know how I got here." He felt bewildered and somewhat depressed. Here he was, his life almost over. Nothing seemed to make sense. The director invited Harry to the center of the group and symbolically walked with him through the times of his life, starting with his first childhood memories. As Harry and the director moved slowly around the group, Harry would fasten on a vivid memory and dramatize a meaningful but long-forgotten experience. He then interacted with group members playing the roles of his parents, siblings, and friends. Some scenes were painful—the death of his mother, losing a job, being wounded in combat. There were also happy memories—the birth of his first child, his first business, and moments with his late wife and grandchildren.

As he moved through these times they came alive to him and revealed patterns and themes he began to connect. In the course of the psychodrama he moved toward the present moment. But having reviewed his life, the present no longer seemed the end of things. Rather, it was a point from which he needed to decide where to go.

In the sharing, other group members discussed their own lives, making connections and gaining perspectives they had not had before. One member had always complained about a business failure that had led to his taking a job with the Post Office and staying there until retirement. Suddenly, he recognized that had he not taken the job, he probably never would have met his wife, with whom he had had many happy years. Another member suggested that Harry contribute skills he had acquired running a catering service to help organize a charity lunch. That way Harry could also meet new people. At the idea of putting his skills to use for a good cause, Harry became excited. He took a long first step toward a productive present and future.

A particular kind of retrospective psychodrama that has proven effective with older group members deals with "unfinished business."

Often individuals find it difficult to concentrate on current life problems because they are caught up in old and seemingly irrevocable
patterns of behavior that leave them feeling hopeless and helpless. It
is as if the individual were motivated by half-forgotten but still emotionally charged conflicts. Sometimes the conflict is so strong that its
manifestations become a dominant theme in the person's life. Whatever the person's real achievements, it remains a source of frustration
and preoccupation. Very often a significant other is the focal point
or embodiment of that "unfinished business."

So it was with Sol, a successful dentist of seventy-one. Sol had
planned for years to retire. He had enough money to do so, but found
himself unable to stop working. He admitted ruefully that he could
not understand how he could both enjoy his work and resent it at the
same time. When he mentioned how much he envied his older brother
Henry, who had made nothing of himself but at least had fun, the
director suspected that there was some unfinished business between
them that needed to be dealt with.

What emerged in the ensuing psychodrama was that Henry had
seemed their mother's secret favorite. While she had scolded Henry
a good deal, she never enforced the punishments she threatened and
Henry did pretty much as he pleased. Although bright and charming,
he never pursued a profession. Instead he traveled widely, involving
himself in farfetched schemes from which his parents often bailed
him out. He had died penniless at a relatively early age.

By contrast, Sol was the "good boy" who followed his mother's
bidding. He always worked hard, trying to win his mother's love by
gaining her approval. She would constantly confide her concern about
Henry to him and would have Sol do Henry's chores so he wouldn't
get in trouble with their father. Sol's mother praised him, but he
always felt that he had to "sing for his supper." He had to produce,
to "be good" in order to get what Henry seemed to command naturally. When Sol grew up, he continued to work hard and became a
respected and prosperous professional, but felt a nagging resentment
and guilt.

In confronting his brother psychodramatically, Sol realized he
was angry as well as jealous. No matter how much a failure Henry
had been, and how successful Sol was, Sol still felt like a loser. Sol
then turned to the group member playing his mother and told her
angrily that he was tired of being a "good boy" and always trying to
please her. Basically a decent person, Sol's feelings about himself were

tainted by his needing to be good. He enjoyed his work but also resented it because he felt he had to produce. If he retired, he wouldn't be "singing for his supper." He feared he would lose his mother's love. As Sol arrived at this realization, he began to cry. But the grief soon gave way to tears of relief and release.

Once Sol had confronted his mother and brother psychodramatically, he felt more prepared to review his current situation and take care of business. He decided that since he enjoyed dentistry, he would continue to do some work in the field. Yet now he was able to engage in the leisure activities he had put off for years because they were only for his own pleasure.

Flora's "unfinished business" was with her dead husband. She described him as a very domineering man who insisted on being in charge of everything. When she encountered him psychodramatically, she first addressed him half-apologetically, saying how lucky she was that he was willing to take on so much responsibility. But as she continued she began to feel anger. She recognized she had tacitly accepted his characterization of her as scatterbrained and incompetent. As a result she had felt inadequate during their entire marriage. She reminded him psychodramatically that she had raised a family and nursed his parents while he was away for four years in the army. Sure, she had been confused and overwhelmed when he had died, but she had taken over running the household. For the first time she admitted, with some relish, that she was relieved he was gone. Although lonely and sometimes depressed, she had never felt so free as she had in the year since he had died.

Then she became aware that she was perpetuating the old image of herself. She was allowing her youngest son, who was still living with her, to order her around as her husband had. Psychodramatically, she confronted her son, stating that while she appreciated his help, she didn't need his controlling behavior. She was competent and capable; if he didn't stop bossing her around, he could leave. Like his father, for all his insistence on control, he needed more taking care of than he ever admitted.

The value of psychodramatic life review and its focus on "unfinished business," then, is that it helps free the protagonist from old conflicts and issues that in one form or another still engage her in the present and limit choices. The result of achieving psychodramatic closure is that the protagonist can now focus more attention and energy on making the last years of life fruitful and productive ones.

Sometimes the issue of "unfinished business" does not require a full-blown psychodrama. It can instead be introduced in a modified form within the group setting. For example, Rebecca began sharing with Flora concerning her own husband, who had insisted that she convert to his religion. The narrative sounded flat until the director suggested that she imagine her husband in an empty chair and speak directly to him. Rebecca did so, expressing with anger that she too felt secretly relieved he was gone so she could choose more freely how she wanted to live her life. The addition of the empty chair and the direction that Rebecca move from descriptive sharing to dialogue helped increase the intensity of her experience.

SOCIODRAMA

Sociodrama is another effective group approach for dealing with significant issues of the elderly. While the psychodrama focuses on problems and interactions emerging from the particular events in the protagonist's life, sociodrama dramatizes and explores themes and situations that are of general interest to the group. Sociodrama is of particular use with newly formed groups. It allows issues of importance to the group to be examined without requiring individuals to expose personal and sensitive events before the group has built up a sufficient level of trust. Sociodrama is a means of sharing on a safer level, while allowing people to participate actively, using their experience and imagination in roles they choose or are assigned.

One way to involve the group in sociodrama is for the therapist to ask for suggestions from different group members concerning themes they might want to explore. Once these are forthcoming, the therapist might ask for recommendations on how to present the issue dramatically. Members then suggest scenes or situations. If several ideas are offered, they may be incorporated into a single sociodrama, or the group may be asked to vote. Sometimes several minidramas are created in one session.

One sociodramatic adaptation is "Where is Sarah?" (Scotto, 1980). An adult daughter, a neighbor, and a social worker are discussing a fictive Sarah, a depressed elderly widow. Sarah was having difficulty shopping and had recently refused to leave the house. She had stopped visiting her social club and going to her social agency for help. The three had the task of deciding whether Sarah should continue to live alone or be put in a nursing home.

Volunteers were elicited from the group to play the neighbor, the daughter and the social worker. The daughter and the neighbor were asked to improvise dialogue voicing their concern for Sarah. The daughter then visited the social worker to discuss her mother. Several group members volunteered to play Sarah. One was defiant and angry, bidding all to go away and leave her alone. A second sat docilely and went along with whatever was suggested. A third approached each player and asked, "What about me? Aren't you concerned with how I feel, or what I want?" When Sarah became angry, her daughter took an apologetic stance. Another group member then asked to play the daughter and started berating her mother for being ungrateful. The social worker was played in a variety of ways, from concerned and caring to hostile and indifferent.

In the discussion that ensued, much anger and frustration was ventilated. Some group members expressed feelings of powerlessness and indignation at not being included in discussions affecting their lives. Some talked of the pressures they felt to act according to their children's ideas of what was good for them, as if with age they had lost the capacity to evaluate their own needs.

Another effective sociodrama uses the theme of generations. It consists of sitting three generations of a make-believe family around the dinner table for a holiday event or family crisis, depending on what is suggested by the group. Different members of the group volunteer to play the various generational roles. Group members then begin to interact with one another according to their own interpretation of the role they are playing. Meanwhile, the group members not directly involved observe the interaction. Sometimes observing group members feel so intensely involved that they ask to participate and speak their piece. Sometimes an interaction between two or three players becomes sufficiently heated or so intense that the director asks the other players to temporarily withdraw and focuses on the interaction.

For example, in a sociodrama depicting a Thanksgiving gathering at an adult daughter's, the group member playing the older adult mother reprimanded her granddaughter for being noisy at the table. At this, her daughter flared up—her mother had no right taking over her role as mother. The granddaughter had every right to act any way she wanted in her own house unless she said otherwise. The director had the other family members withdraw. In the interchange between mother and adult daughter, questions of responsibility, authority, and respect for each other's roles arose.

After an initial heated interaction, discussion between the players ensued. Then the other group members were asked to comment on what they observed, or to share from their own experiences, both as adult children with their parents and as older adults with their own adult children. The general group feedback was that both mother and daughter needed to look at their behavior. The older adult had to stop automatically assuming the authority role and to defer to her daughter in her own house. For her part, the daughter needed to be less defensive, always experiencing her mother as critical of her ability to act appropriately as a mother.

Other group members asked to play either the older adult or her daughter. In these roles, they offered alternative interactions. One member took the granddaughter's role and criticized both her mother and her grandmother for their rigid positions. Sometimes an impasse was avoided by having the opposing players reverse roles and try to experience the situation from the other's point of view. Other ways for breaking impasses were sought by different group members. In the older role, one relieved tension by saying, "Being a mother is not easy; I'm proud of you." Another admitted to her daughter that she was so used to jumping in she had forgotten herself. A third, as the adult daughter, said, "I get so upset because it's important to me for you to see I can be a good mother too." If time permits, the family group might be reassembled around the holiday table to continue until another theme emerges.

Sometimes sociodramas shade off into role training. In role training, group members examine practical issues with which they may be having difficulty. The role training is used as a laboratory as they attempt various behaviors in particular situations in order to discover an effective approach. Others in the group help by giving feedback regarding a member's effectiveness. For example, one elderly group member wanted to present a sociodrama of visiting the doctor. What ensued was a sometimes serious, sometimes comic interaction. One doctor was depicted as standing on a chair looking down at the older adult, who was sitting like a small child on the floor. Another doctor was played as an ogre who kept muttering, "if you don't stop asking me questions, I'll tell you something you'll be sorry to hear." The group members initially enjoyed ventilating some of their fears and frustrations.

One group member raised the issue of not knowing how to act in a medical setting so as to be taken seriously, not seen simply as an old pest who complains a lot. What ensued was a role training session in which a group member first played his doctor. Then he tried various ways of acting in relation to the doctor to get the attention and service he wanted. Finally he found a way which felt comfortable and seemed effective, at least in the group interaction. During the exploration he was able to stop the action to deal with feelings that were inhibiting his behavior. Other group members gave him feedback as to how he was coming across. Group members with similar problems then experimented with different approaches.

In subsequent groups, members shared their experiences in actual life situations. When they hadn't been effective, they tried to reexamine what had happened and to change their behavior. In one instance Rhoda, a seventy-three-year-old widow, had been intimidated by her doctor before "speaking up to him" in a role training session. She was then able to overcome his real-life discounting of her aching knee without so much as examining it. "After all," was his attitude, "as one gets older, one has to expect some discomfort in the joints." She had pointed out that her other knee was equally old, but not hurting. How could he account for that? Upon examination, he found that she had in fact strained a ligament and needed some attention.

Implicit in role training is a recognition of real changes which have occurred to the individual as a result of old age. Yet there is a significant countermeasure against age stereotyping built into the exercises, particularly those involving encounters with professionals such as doctors, lawyers, and social workers. The older adults also become more sensitive to the self-stereotyping revealed in their tacit acceptance of the limiting and demeaning images others may project onto them.

In the role training work, group members have explicit permission to ask for help, thereby admitting openly that they need it and have the right to seek it. Sometimes help is needed with problems of daily living, such as shopping, or maintaining an apartment. But in the process of exposing and exploring these needs, the group members are also recognizing that the problems they are raising are not unsolvable; they can still learn new approaches and practical alternatives to old behaviors.

In the sharing of mutual concerns, which occurs throughout but most directly at the end of a group session, members often experience a sense of closeness and community. Through the exploration of feelings elicited by their activities, group members undergo major changes in attitude. They move from a sense of desperate groping with life under reduced capacities and fewer opportunities to the experience of solving concrete problems. Difficulties and life stresses that have appeared overwhelming now seem more manageable for having been shared.

REFERENCES

Aiken, L. R. (1982), *Later Life*, 2nd ed. New York: Holt, Rinehart & Winston.
Altman, K. P. (1983), Psychodrama with the institutionalized elderly: A method for role re-engagement. *J. Group Psychother., Psychodrama & Sociometry*, 36(3):87–94.
Brody, E. M. (1973), Aging and family personality: A developmental view. *Family Process*, 11:23–37.
———— (1979), Aging. In: *Encyclopedia of Social Work*, Vol. 1. Washington, DC: National Association of Social Workers, pp. 713–718.
Buchanan, D. R. (1981), Psychodrama: A humanistic approach to psychiatric treatment for the elderly. *Hospital & Community Psychiat.*, 33:220–223.
Cumming, E., & Dean, L. R. (1972), Disengagement: A tentative theory of aging. In: *Human Aging*, ed. S. M. Chown. Baltimore: Penguin Books, pp. 269–283.
Erikson, E. (1980), *Childhood and Society*. New York: Norton.
Nissenson, M. (1984), Therapy after sixty. *Psychology Today*, 26:22–26.
Preston, S. H. (1984), Children and the elderly in the U.S. *Scientific American*, 251(6):44–49.
Scotto, A. (1980), Helping friends and neighbors. *Aging & Mental Health: Brooklyn White House Conference*, 16:1–6.
Uhlenberg, P. (1979), Older women: The growing challenge to design constructive roles. *Gerontologist*, 19:236–241.

Part III

Supportive/Rehabilitative
Group Therapy in the Community

7

Group Psychotherapy with Geriatric Outpatients: A Model for Treatment and Training

SUSAN MATORIN, M.S., A.C.S.W. and
BORIS ZOUBOK, M.D.

STRUCTURE AND FORMAT

The psychotherapeutic group described here was initiated in a traditional outpatient psychiatric clinic within a major teaching hospital. The group, comprising seven members, was formed by a psychiatry resident and the senior staff social worker. Members were recruited from cohorts of clinic patients treated in individual psychotherapy or medication clinics by psychiatry residents who were rotating off service and in the process of transferring their caseloads. Selection was guided by only two inclusion criteria: patients had to be in need of continued treatment and had to be over sixty-five. The group was started in the context of a major clinic reorganization emphasizing group psychotherapy as an important treatment modality for chronic patients. Many of these patients had been carried by the clinic for years and had been accustomed to brief monthly contact with a psychiatric resident, never having the same doctor for more than six months or a year. Charts of all patients referred to this group were carefully reviewed, and with most patients the nature of group therapy was discussed by both leaders. All patients who entered the group consented to this form of treatment, though for most of them, not without feelings of uneasiness. Curiously enough, they shared the basis of their fears more freely with some of the clerical staff: loss of a direct patient-doctor relationship, and fears of exposure to intolerant group members.

The initial goal of the group was to create a supportive environment and provide a socialization experience for elderly clinic patients. A commonality of experience was assumed. It was our belief that the group would provide a supportive network in which to develop and enhance patients' coping skills so as to alleviate symptoms of psychological distress—anxiety, fears, insomnia, etc.—and decrease social isolation (Berger and Berger, 1973)

Group meetings were always held in the same room and became a rather set routine. Tea was served, we sat in a circle, and patients alternated bringing in refreshments, often homemade. This created an atmosphere of warmth and familiarity. We believe that over time this gave our patients a sense of security that facilitated psychotherapeutic exploration.

Arranging the group as a social event, at least in appearance, set the tone for concerned and caring attitudes toward one another which developed quickly among the membership. When one member, Florinda M. (see Table 7.1), became acutely ill and had to be operated on, the entire group seized on this opportunity to have a meeting by her bedside. Florinda still spoke of this a year later, describing it as "the best medicine" she had received. When another patient was hospitalized with the prospect of major cardiac surgery, telephone calls to her husband and get-well cards became part of the group process.

In its first year the group met once a month, always in the latter part of the morning, as patients quickly informed us that an early morning time was taxing and stressful. In the second year patients were invited to meet every other week. The more active members of the group agreed to do so: others elected to attend only monthly. This flexibility allowed some members to maintain a comfortable distance from the group process and thereby enhanced their sense of independence. While therapeutically sound, this same flexibility presented technical difficulties for the leaders, as continuity of theme from meeting to meeting was occasionally disrupted. We tried to deal with this problem by actively developing a therapeutic focus within each meeting, or by making brief reports, at the beginning of each session, on the content of the previous meeting and the nature of our phone contacts with group members who were unable to attend. This way of dealing with the inevitable disruption of the group process became an important part of the structure of meetings.

TABLE 7.1

Name/Age	Ethnicity/ Religion	Psychiatric Diagnosis DSM–III	Medical Diagnosis	Psych Meds	Occupation and Social Situation	Psycho- social Stressors	GAS Scores Initial	Current
F.M.-66	White, Hispanic, Catholic	Dysthymic Disorder	s/p Cholescystectomy Hypertension	Librium 10 mg Tid	Lives with husband, daughter, & grandson	Family Stress	51	65
J.R.-84	White, Jewish	Generalized Anxiety Disorder	Legally blind, Hearing impair. Cor. Heart Disease	none	Lives alone	Physical Dis. Loneliness	61	65
S.H.-60	Black, Catholic	s/p Grief Reaction Adjustment Dis. with depressed mood. Mixed Personality Disorder	Aortic Valve Disease s/p Stroke, Hyperten- sion, Obesity	Ativan 1 mg Bid	with spouse	Loss of 2 Siblings, Medical Illness	71	51
E.M.-85	Black, Protestant	Adjustment Dis. with depressed mood. Senile Dementia	Conduction Disorder, Diabetes	None	Retired Cook Widow	Aging Care for elderly ill spouse	65	60
A.F.-75	White, Irish, Catholic	Dysthymic Disorder	Glaucoma, Irrit. Bowel Syn., Sensorineural Hearing Loss, Stress Incontinence	None	Retired Sec'y Lives with spouse	Deaths of 2 children	65	70

(continued)

TABLE 7.1 (Continued)

							Avg. GAS initial x̄ = 58	Avg. GAS current x̄ = 61
M.S.-79	Black, Baptist	Paranoid Personality Disorder, Somatization Disorder	Arthritis, Vision Impairment	None	"Floats" Among Children	?	65	60
R.P.-72	Black, Unitarian	Paranoia	—	None	Housekeeper Currently Employed	Aging	51	75
A.F.-70	White, Irish, Catholic	Dysthymic Disability Alcohol Abuse Mixed Personality	Eczema, Irritable bowel, Bilateral Cataracts	Dalmane 15 mg Hs	Retired Legal Sec'y—lives solo	Loneliness	60	60
E.K.-72 (sister)	White, Jewish	Retardation, Moderate Mixed Personality	CHF	Haldol 5 mg Hs	with sister (institutionalized)	Organic Brain Disease	31	40
M.G.-80	White, Jewish	s/p Grief Reaction Mixed Personality	Obesity	None	Retired Sec'y Lives alone	Loss of sib. Loneliness	60	61
Avg. age x̄ = 74 yrs								

Originally only identified patients participated in the group. When it became obvious that a husband of one of the patients was regularly accompanying her to meetings and patiently sitting in the waiting area of the clinic, we decided to invite him to join the group. Thus a precedent was set; since that time, two other spouses were welcomed into the group, and later the sister of one of our patients. This allowed us to make family interventions and to extend the treatment well beyond our original goal of providing a socialization experience. During the second year of our work the nature of the group changed noticeably: from our initial focus on socialization we arrived at a situation in which inquiries into psychological motivation were initiated by the patients themselves. Not only were group members tolerating exploratory and interpretive comments from us, but some were making rather astute and perceptive comments to one another.

But once psychological motivation and the meaning of behaviors and life choices became the group's focus, we were confronted by the inability of some members to tolerate the anxiety engendered by discussion of such issues as death, physical disability, loneliness, and sexual behavior in old age. The presence of two leaders allowed us to split and alternate roles: when one of us was supportive and tolerant of expressed anger, the other could maintain an interpretive posture and the freedom to set limits and, occasionally, to confront disruptive behavior or avoidance (Foster and Foster, 1983; Spitz, 1984). Moreover, the strain of dealing with affectively charged material—most specifically the necessary themes of loss, death, and fear of dying—became more tolerable when shared with a coleader. All members of the group maintained a highly respectful attitude toward us and only rarely were critical. They chose to call us by our last names—"You earned the title *Doctor*"—but agreed to use first names among themselves and asked us to do the same.

THEMES AND PROCESS

Acceptance of aging and physical disability, and adaptation to it, emerged early as a principal theme. Jeanette R., a petite, frail, but sprightly woman of eighty-four who was legally blind, almost deaf, walked with a cane, and lived alone, was referred to us by a medical social worker after the patient had repeatedly threatened suicide. For years Jeanette had managed quite well using the resources of the Guild for the Blind and jealously guarding her independence from her two daughters. During evaluation and in her first group meetings, she spoke forcefully of her rage at insensitive ophthalmologists who gave her ill-fitting glasses, and her troubles with a variety of dentists who tried to convince her to wear dentures. Clearly the patient experienced a recent deterioration in her vision as a major threat to her independence. In subsequent meetings it became clear that she viewed dentures as a symbol of old age.

Sadie H., while the youngest of the group, had the most severe medical problems. She was referred to us after brief treatment for a grief reaction following the death of two siblings, and a miraculous recovery from a massive stroke. An obese woman who looked much older than her age, she clutched her cane and was reluctant to stand or walk without her husband's support. She had obvious difficulty in keeping up her appearance and relied on the women in her extended family to help her. Right from the start the patient was torn between a need to take medication that would reduce her anxiety and her fears of "becoming a junkie." Only over time could she reluctantly let the group know her secret—she lived in constant dread that "nerves" or the slightest exertion would bring on another stroke and leave her a "living vegetable." In her fear she experienced her body as her enemy and described it as a "time bomb."

Belle R. (no longer a member of the group), a sixty-eight-year-old retired nurse who lost her only son to a tragic and sudden death, was one of our original and most active members. Very obese, she suffered from extensive arthritis which kept her in constant and ever-increasing pain. She suffered also from diabetes, hypertension, and disseminated and recurrent skin rashes. Despite feelings of shame about her obesity, she took considerable care with her appearance and was never without jewelry and perfume. Her unending grief over the loss of her son made her shy away from contact with old friends and even her attentive daughter-in-law and grandsons. Her physical condition and limited financial resources severely restricted her lifestyle. She described herself as "a young person trapped in an old body."

Essie K., a tall, stately eighty-five-year-old retired cook, was referred to us by her internist, who described her as despondent and anxious. This patient was very active and assertive all her life and stopped working well past usual retirement age because of progressive weakness; she made the care of a cantankerous and severely demented husband the center of her life. Over time, with her own age advancing, feeling weaker and more forgetful, she became increasingly incapable of caring for her husband; yet she adamantly refused to dip into their life's savings to purchase more home care service or nursing home placement. For as long as she could care for him she could deny her own aging and developing disability, thereby maintaining self-esteem. Once she could no longer ignore her weakness, she started feeling overburdened and became depressed, seeing in her husband her own future.

The group responded to each of these life situations by rallying around these patients, and allowing them to express their feelings of fear, despondency, and rage. This would occur in an atmosphere of accepting silence. Immediately following, other members would describe similar feelings and experiences. Only after the commonality of experience was established, one or another member (usually the same people) would restate the experience in positive terms, emphasizing hope and coping strengths. In the first few instances the leaders had to take a very active role to stimulate and maintain this process; after several recurrences, the group would respond spontaneously to any similar experience of threat to function. The outcome of this process was most dramatic in Essie's case. This patient, who before joining our group was thought to have a major depression, and was treated with antidepressants and worked up for possible ECT, improved so rapidly and markedly that all medications were discontinued.

In the second six months of the group, we accepted Bessie B., a remarkable Russian Jewish woman of eighty-one. She was severely disabled by paralysis following removal of a brain tumor thirty years ago, and was now demoralized and suicidal over increasing loss of ambulation. Her psychological state at this point compromised rehabilitation efforts. The patient, frail and decrepit, slumped in a wheelchair and held a cup of tea tremulously. Considerable work by the leaders was necessary to integrate her because she represented to everyone in the group, in a very concrete way, the physical deterioration that often accompanies old age. At this stage of group development, members did not visit her during her hospitalization a year later, the final days of her life. They were able, however, to appreciate her courage, her extraordinary thirst for life, and helped her share fears of increased dependency and despondency. Her death was the first in our group. Members did not directly grieve her because they had emotionally distanced themselves from this frail woman; nonetheless her loss was experienced as a very immediate threat to the group's continuity. Members raised concerned questions about the status of Dr. Zoubok in the group and the predictable change of coleader at the end of the academic year. It was at this point that we realized that the group had become a lifeline and support system for our patients.

Particularly during discussions of loss and death, we noticed in the last year and a half that members seemed to have settled into very specific roles: some would identify in an empathic way with painful feelings of grief and guilt, allowing a person reporting a tragic loss to fully express these feelings; others, finding such discussions painful and intolerable, would attempt to refocus the group's attention on a more hopeful topic; still others would always cap the discussion by underscoring the courage to survive and endure. To illustrate, Alice F., a seventy-five-year-old devout Irish Catholic who lost both of her children in infancy, was encouraged by us to talk about the events surrounding their deaths. Because she was not allowed to ride in the ambulance with one of her dying daughters, she lived with guilt that this child had "died in the streets of New York without her mother." Her husband revealed that they had never before shared that with each other. Listening to Alice, we all felt overwhelming grief, as if these losses had just occurred. Sadie H. helped Alice label her pain as guilt. Another member responded by calling the discussion "too painful," reminding the group that "we are here to get better." With only a gentle reminder from the leaders that the group meets to share all kinds of feelings, this member grasped Alice's hand and told her how strong she was to have lived through this loss, and how lucky she was to have a husband in her old age. Thus we learned to rely on different members to raise disturbing issues, to modulate group responses, and to balance the impact of painful losses with optimism and reaffirmation of strengths (Berland and Poggi, 1979). As discussion of such issues generated a fair degree of tension, we sometimes extended sessions to allow the process to complete itself.

Members of the group came from a wide variety of ethnic and religious backgrounds. Religious identification played an important role in the lives of all our patients, and when they began to share this we took it as evidence of group cohesion. Many times hope was stated in religious terms and faith invoked to counter suicidal ideas and relieve feelings of despair. During the holiday season, Christians and Jews in the group educated each other about their faiths and discussed the meaning of festivities. Sadie H., the group's voice of tolerance and empathy, expressed everyone's feeling when she stated that a belief in God unites members and makes denominational differences less relevant. Reever P., a seventy-two-year-old black woman, elegant and staunchly independent, emphasized the role of faith in overcoming difficulties. Employed as a housekeeper for a silk-stocking would-be politician, she presented with a florid paranoid delusion encapsulated from her otherwise high functional abilities. Initially guarded, tense, and rigid in her belief that an upstairs neighbor was deliberately torturing her with laser beams and electrical waves directed to her body, she baffled the group, who had never before been exposed to a psychotic thought disorder. This woman, who always before had refused medication, accepted it for the first time in the group setting as a means to "strengthen her" in her battle with this persecutor. She also started to rely more heavily on prayer to the same end; when her condition improved on Haldol, she accepted this as evidence of the efficacy of faith. Since that time she has used this experience to encourage others in crisis to pray similarly. Rather than confront her denial of the role of medication, we allowed her to maintain her self-esteem with the assertion that her lifelong belief system had protected her. Reever P. frequently reads passages from the Bible to others in distress—for the group an acceptable way to respond to crisis.

"PROBLEM MEMBERS"

During the lifetime of the group we failed to integrate two patients. Despite the cohesion of the group we were unable to engage Bessie G. at the time of her introduction. This seventy-six-year-old retired Jewish lady, clearly lonely and isolated, concealed dependency needs and despair over increasing loss of vision with sharp, sarcastic, and vituperative behavior (see Levine and Poston, 1980). This behavior had resulted in her extrusion from available senior centers in her neighborhood. She presented herself at her first meeting with an entry ticket—homemade muffins—symbolic of her desire to be accepted. Refused by one member on a diet, Bessie defended against this blow to her fragile self-esteem by countering with a verbal assault on the dieting patient, criticizing her inability to maintain a diet as due to "pure laziness," and challenging the relevance of a group discussion of weight control to psychotherapy. In the few subsequent meetings she attended, the group was unable to tolerate her provocative behavior, which included sitting on the sidelines outside the group circle and verbal attacks on the leaders. On one occasion, and in the presence of a black member (Mabel S.), Bessie alluded to a deterioration of her apartment building due to an increase in minority tenants. Mabel dramatically turned her chair away from the circle but was otherwise unable to express herself. Bessie became enraged when we attempted to protect Mabel by suggesting the offensiveness of the remark. (This was in fact the only occasion on which racial issues surfaced.) Subsequently, when the physician coleader was absent, this patient stormed out of the group and tore up her clinic payment receipt, refusing to attend a group without the "doctor present." Our efforts to create an empathic environment for her, so as to explore her underlying loneliness and fears while setting limits on her disdain, were unsuccessful, and she withdrew from the group after several months.

It is noteworthy that while we were unable to engage this patient over the long term, in point of fact her verbalization of negative affect advanced the group process. While members were clearly upset by her criticism of the leaders, their ability to interact with her was significant. For example, the patient shared her history of unresolved anger at her mother for ruining her life, interfering with romantic opportunities, etc. This was expressed with such venom that we had difficulty remembering that the mother was long deceased. At a later point, as the patient described many negative interactions with nursing staff during a hospital stay, group members made an astute transference interpretation. Similarly, the patient had numerous complaints about lack of attention from her only brother; group members attempted to clarify reasonable expectations for sibling involvement. (At this point in the group process the leaders had difficulty remembering the group's origins as a socialization experience.) In retrospect we believe that one of the reasons for Bessie's rejection by the group was her focused attack on a beloved group member who was by then acting as a spokesperson for group feelings.

Another ejected patient was Iago L., a seventy-two-year-old research biochemist who was referred to us because of depression following his mandatory retirement from a major university. He came to his first meeting carrying an attaché case and a copy of the *Wall Street Journal.* Clearly avoiding the group, he immediately tried to engage the physician coleader in a private conversation using one of the many foreign languages in which he was fluent. Right from the start, despite his expressed intention "just to sit and listen," he quickly monopolized group time. In a very ostentatious way and using elaborate vocabulary interspersed with French phrases, he addressed his lengthy remarks to the male coleader, excluding the rest of the group. He ignored all attempts by other members to genuinely empathize with his despondency over loss of his job—so central to his life and self-esteem—and his fruitless efforts to obtain other employment. As always, this issue united the entire group in expressing angry feelings toward a society that discards its elderly people prematurely. Our group members, most with histories of responsible skilled employment but lacking the financial resources or physical health to enjoy the "fruits of retirement," articulated the loss of self-esteem, further isolation, and limited income that now defined their lives. Feeling rebuffed by Iago, the group switched from a supportive and understanding posture to an angry and critical one. After only three meetings Iago withdrew.

CONCLUSION

We believe that group psychotherapy with elderly patients is an invaluable training experience for all disciplines involved in providing mental health care. Generic skills are needed because of the complexities of comprehensive care for a geriatric population. This involves specific knowledge about health and disease in old age, and of the many socioeconomic pressures that compound the stressors of aging. The self-esteem of elderly persons is assaulted daily by shrinking sources of gratification—the loss of loved ones, physical disability, forced retirement, and inevitable exposure to an insensitive medical care system. The group format provides a safe and appropriate arena in which feelings of anger and despondency can be expressed and explored so that dysfunctional and maladaptive behavior can be modified and coping skills reinforced (Berland and Poggi, 1979). Group process should be focused on functioning and responses to stress rather than symptomatology. As group interaction brings attention to the talents, hobbies, and political views of different members, and as news items are discussed and holidays celebrated, models for successful adaptation become available (Williams, 1979). The process itself, through its relentless continuity, encourages patients to function to their fullest capacity with regard to daily life activity and social contacts. Once this process is established, a more impaired patient can be integrated into the group without major disruption.

The evaluation of outcome measures has troubled us throughout (Coche and Dies, 1981; Parham, Priddy, McGovern, and Richman, 1982). We have included initial and current GAS scores in Table 7.1. The scores of many of the members have improved slightly, which would be considered a positive outcome for this age group (Liederman, Green, and Liederman, 1967). Since it has been suggested that elderly patients utilize medical clinics and emergency rooms in search of social contact beyond actual treatment needs for physical symptoms, tracking such visits over time with a hypothesized decrease would be valuable additional data (Paradis, 1973; Deutsch and Kramer, 1977). We do not feel confident, however, that such measures accurately reflect the major changes we have noted in self-esteem regulation and the development of assertive and adaptive behavior.

To illustrate: Esther K., a seventy-two-year-old moderately retarded patient with a history of lifelong institutionalization joined the group with her sister, a spunky eighty-three-year-old. Overburdened by her decision to bring the patient home, the sister was critical, irritable, and clearly mortified by the patient's inappropriate behavior in public. At the initial contact the patient was mute and withdrawn. The sister literally screeched her anxiety at the leaders. In two years of monthly contact, however, the pair blossomed: the identified patient assisted in arranging chairs for each meeting, listened attentively, asked appropriate questions, shared in household chores, and clearly responded to the increased approval she received from members for the crafts she produced and brought in. The caretaking sister, who initially allowed no one to directly engage the patient, and attended only because of the patient, obviously benefited from the support and acknowledgment by group members of her altruistic behavior. She participated actively in discussions of politics, reminiscences, etc. and decreased her own sense of isolation by regularly taking the patient to concerts.

Most important, such change measures as noted above fail to reflect the courage, effort, and ego strengths of our patients which they muster to struggle with chronic pain, frequent losses, inflation, and compromised personal safety. Throughout our work we were impressed by the many untapped abilities of our patients, which now cannot find expression because of retirement and social isolation.

We have had to overcome our own prejudices concerning the possibilities of engaging elderly persons in active and rewarding therapeutic work. For a psychodynamically oriented professional in training to learn to respond to a deaf person who disrupts group process by switching seats, so as to be near the speaker and feel included, was no small task. Confronting our own fears of aging and loss of function, and our immediate concerns about aging parents and grandparents, is even more difficult and anxiety-provoking. An opportunity to observe first-hand the interface of psychological, social, and physical stress with a rigid structure of defenses at a later stage of the life cycle is important in mental health training. The recent extension of longevity makes such training mandatory (Ross, 1975).

Elderly people, so sadly familiar with impatience, disinterest, and rebuff, are genuinely grateful for the therapist's interest and concern. It is rare in clinical work that one can unquestionably accept such open appreciation for what it is, without interpretation.

REFERENCES

Berger, L. F., & Berger, M. M. (1973), A holistic group approach to psychogeriatric outpatients. *Internat. J. Group Psychother.*, 23:432–444.

Berland, D. I., & Poggi, R. (1979), Expressive group psychotherapy with the aging. *Internat. J. Group Psychother.*, 29:87–108.

Coche, E., & Dies, R. R. (1981), Integrating research findings into the practice of group psychotherapy. *Psychotherapy: Theory, Research & Practice*, 18:410–416.

Deutsch, C. B., & Kramer, N. (1977), Outpatient group psychotherapy for the elderly: An alternative to institutionalization. *Hospital & Community Psychiat.*, 28:440–442.

Foster, J. R., & Foster, R. P. (1983), Group therapy with the old and aged. In: *Comprehensive Group Psychotherapy: Vol. II*, ed. H. I. Kaplan & B. Sadock. Baltimore: Williams & Wilkins, pp. 269–278.

Levine, B. E., & Poston, M. (1980), A modified group treatment for elderly narcissistic patients. *Internat. J. Group Psychother.*, 30:153–167.

Liederman, P., Green, R., & Liederman, V. (1967), OPD group therapy with geriatric patients. *Geriatrics*, 22:148–153.

Paradis, A. P. (1973), Brief outpatient group psychotherapy with older patients in the treatment of age-related problems. *Dissertation Abstracts Internat.*, 34:2947B.

Parham, I. A., Priddy, J. M., McGovern, T. V., & Richman, C. M. (1982), Group psychotherapy with the elderly: Problems and prospects. *Psychotherapy: Theory, Research & Practice*, 19:437–443.

Ross, M. (1975), A review of some recent group psychotherapy methods for elderly psychiatric patients. In: *Community Geriatric Group Therapies: A Comprehensive Review*, ed. M. Rosenbaum & M. Berger. New York: Basic Books.

Spitz, H. I. (1984), Contemporary trends in group psychotherapy: A literature survey. *Hospital & Community Psychiat.*, 35:132–142.

Williams, C. L. (1979), Nurse therapist high empathy and nurse therapist low empathy during therapeutic group work as factors in changing the self-concept of the institutionalized aged. *Dissertation Abstracts Internat.*, 40:3095B.

8

Activity Group Psychotherapy for the Inner-City Elderly

DANIEL B. FISHER, M.D., Ph.D.

The elderly of our society are increasingly isolated and alienated. Age segregation, urban renewal, increased mobility, and ageism have each contributed to this phenomenon. The trend is especially true for the inner-city elderly who find themselves without family or friends to support them. As this segment of our population grows in proportion to working adults, we will need to devise new strategies for maintaining their autonomy and dignity as long as is feasible, while they live in their homes. Several factors have limited our capacity to serve these needs. Home care organizations have addressed the housekeeping and nutritional needs of many elderly at risk of institutionalization. These organizations, however, have rarely addressed the social and emotional needs of this population. Community mental health centers have attempted to meet their emotional needs. Unfortunately, the elderly do not use these services because they still tend to believe that people who see psychotherapists must be crazy. Furthermore, few mental health clinics are accessible and affordable to the elderly. Medicare provides only two hundred fifty dollars a year in coverage for outpatient psychotherapy. In addition, Medicare guidelines for the provision of such therapy are very restrictive. Medicare requires that

a psychiatrist provide all services and that these conform to a traditional model of psychotherapy. Since a majority of geriatric therapists
are not psychiatrists and the traditional model of psychotherapy is
less appropriate for the elderly, these Medicare guidelines make it
very difficult to fund outpatient psychotherapy for the poor elderly
through third-party sources.

During five years of experience (1978–1983) at the Outlook Clinic
for the Elderly, it was found that group psychotherapy which includes
an activity is an appropriate and effective technique for combating
the isolation and alienation of the inner-city elderly. This finding
corresponds with that of Birren and Sloane (1980), who have pointed
out that group psychotherapy with the elderly which incorporates an
activity is often more useful than groups which are only verbal. They
call this type of therapy activity group psychotherapy, which differs
from recreational activity groups "by its therapeutic focus characterized by the use of verbal and nonverbal expressions for approaching
the problems felt by the group members. . . ." (pp. 818–822). Reichenfield, Csapo, Carriere, and Gardner (1973) found that activity
group psychotherapy decreased the hostility and behavioral deterioration of patients on a geropsychiatric unit. Blackman, Howe, and
Pinkston (1976) found that this approach improved the social interaction among the institutionalized elderly. In this chapter we will
describe the development and delivery of activity psychotherapy
groups at the Outlook Clinic.

ACTIVITY PSYCHOTHERAPY GROUPS CONDUCTED BY THE OUTLOOK CLINIC

History of the Outlook Clinic

The Outlook Clinic was founded in 1978 as a geropsychiatry
program to provide therapy to the elderly in their homes. The clinic
was initially funded by a three-year grant from the Administration
on Aging, HHS. The purpose of the clinic was to demonstrate the
efficacy of individual and group psychotherapy in reducing the rate
of institutionalization of an at-risk elderly population. A survey of the
clients seen during the first two years of the clinic revealed they had
little contact with their families. Fewer than half the clients had living
children and of these fewer than one-fourth saw their children weekly.
In addition, only 12 percent of the clients had contact with some other
relative (Leiff, 1984). Since families provide a majority of home care

support (Butler and Lewis, 1982), our clients were at high risk of institutionalization.

Groups Created at the Clinic

Though the majority of the service was individual psychotherapy, a few groups were started during the clinic's first two years. The leaders first tried to engage clients in verbal groups of the type developed for young adults. The majority of elderly clients quickly dropped out of these verbal groups, with the complaint that they didn't see the point of getting together just to talk.

In order to meet the clients' requests, we incorporated a variety of activities into our groups. The activity modalities utilized in these groups were arts and crafts, food preparation, music, and exercise. In 1981, in response to a 75 percent reduction in budget, the clinic shifted completely to a group program.

Supervision and Training of Group Leaders

During the first two years, groups were led by therapists experienced in interpersonal dynamics and one of the activities utilized. Supervision was provided in a group format by a psychologist. Subsequently, each group was co-led by a psychiatrist and an assistant while supervision was provided by the psychiatrist in a group format. The training of group leaders was an ongoing process provided by the supervision, the actual group experience, case conferences, and reading assignments. A constant challenge in supervision was how to enable the group leaders to adequately balance the interpersonal and activity orientations. One group leader, with more extensive experience in teaching sculpture than in group dynamics, tended to overemphasize the production of a finished piece at the expense of encouraging group process. Another group leader tended to get overinvolved in discussion at the expense of the organized activity. Each responded well to feedback in the supervision group.

General Principles for Creating Successful Groups

By the third year of the clinic, certain principles had emerged which characterized successful groups. The goal of each group was described to the clients as being to provide a forum in which to discuss problems of common interest to their neighbors—crime, loneliness, frustrations with the housing authority (most group members were residents of public housing).

It was important to select members based on their sharing the same neighborhood and similar emotional problems. A great majority of the group members suffered from varying degrees of depression due to multiple losses. To combat this depression it was necessary for the group leaders to be highly motivated and optimistic regarding the potential of each member. The group format in supervision was essential in maintaining staff morale, as staff cohesion and mutual support combats burnout and discouragement. Group leaders were left free to devise their own means of interweaving group discussion and group activity. The two major approaches were either to divide the group into forty-five minutes of activity and forty-five minutes of discussion or to stop action and discuss points as they arise in the activity.

Therapeutic Nutrition Groups as Examples of Activity Group Psychotherapy

To combine the most valuable aspects of group psychotherapy and meal sites we started several therapeutic nutrition groups in public housing community rooms which had been unable to sustain meal sites. We were asked to run these groups by the housing managers because in addition to lacking a meal site they had also lost their social workers due to cutbacks in housing authority funds in 1981.

Residents were referred to the group leaders by the housing manager or other group members. A group leader would interview each prospective member to determine how necessary the group was and to describe the operation of the group to them. Some residents needed a number of brief meetings with a group leader before they were sufficiently secure and motivated to attend the group. Those who did attend helped each week in menu selection and food preparation, thereby experiencing greater control over their environment. This improved their motivation and self-esteem. The group members shared isolation as a major problem. One year 80 percent of the group members were not invited by family or friends for Thanksgiving dinner.

The nutrition groups acted primarily as surrogate families to help members combat loneliness and consequent depression. The main task of the leaders was to foster cohesion among the members. The first stage of that process involved overcoming the mistrust that members felt based on negative experiences of the past. In addition to the managers' assistance, we also gained trust by working closely with the other important people in the members' lives: guards, maintenance men, and homemakers. Even more important, we leaders had to show the members that we were trustworthy by showing that we cared about their welfare, that we could listen to them, that we were consistent, and that we treated them with respect.

Once some trust was established, the members showed a high degree of dependence on the leaders. For a while they expected us to make most of the important decisions about the group. When we pointed out this trend to the members, and asked that they share the running of the group with us, they got angry. At that point we became the target of the bottled-up rage that members had felt toward parents and other authorities in the past. When they ventilated their anger and saw that the leaders stayed with them, a deeper trust and cooperation developed. After that, the members participated in group problem solving and developed a greater sense of cohesion.

Once the members felt part of a secure group they were able to express aggressive and sexual feelings toward one another. In one group, a seventy-five-year-old man wheeled a cart in front of a fifty-nine-year-old woman who was using a walker. "Why don't you watch where you are going!" she yelled at him. "You're not going to yell at me!" he shouted back, with raised fist. They exchanged more harsh words, while the rest of the group silently watched. The leaders got the two to talk out the episode. Though neither was willing to apologize, tempers ran their course. After incidents such as this, both participants and onlookers usually said it was good to get some anger "off their chests," that "it livens up the dead place." Sexual feelings were usually expressed through jokes. It took a while for the leaders, whose ages ranged from twenty-two to thirty-nine, to feel comfortable hearing bawdy jokes from the elderly members. But once we got to know them better we became more accepting and could see the jokes as helping to liven up the group.

The members also felt freer to give mutual assistance to one another. For example, a seventy-nine-year-old Lebanese woman had developed such a severe tremor that she was unable to unlock her door. A seventy-two-year-old black woman whom she met in the group started regularly to accompany her upstairs to unlock her door. Other members are frequently puzzled by notices they receive in the mail. An articulate eighty-four-year-old member overcame her possessiveness and invited a social worker from another agency to explain one of these letters to the group. The members also provide positive feedback to one another. A sixty-nine-year-old woman had a long history of epilepsy. For this she had been ridiculed in the past. She secretly confided in one of the leaders that she was sure the other members didn't like her. Consequently, she rarely talked to others. Then, at the start of one group, she had a minor seizure. Though she soon recovered, she was very ashamed. Contrary to her expectations, however, the other members were supportive and empathetic. In each subsequent session she was more comfortable in the group and participated more freely.

Although the members were lively and enjoyed the company of younger people, we were able to introduce students only after the group had developed sufficient cohesion and trust. The students were then welcomed as new faces and new life in these age-segregated settings. For the students, the groups provided an opportunity to get to know elderly persons outside the hospital setting. Medical students in the first two years of their studies have learned interviewing techniques in a natural manner.

The nutrition groups played an important role in strengthening an informal peer support network. In contrast to traditional psychotherapy groups, which discourage contact among members outside the group setting, we encouraged such contact. We also invited informal caregivers and family to join the groups so they could get to know the members better. This had the added benefit of allowing the professional leaders to train these informal caregivers through imitation and discussion. Similarly, the members themselves learned more effective means of helping each other by observing the professional leaders. In both groups, the informal caregivers and members started to identify the most needy residents and invite them to the group.

In summary, our therapeutic nutrition groups provided the interpersonal learning, the trust building, the expression of feelings, and the resolution of conflicts found in verbal psychotherapy groups. They also provided informal social support and nutritious meals.

EXAMPLES OF INDIVIDUALS HELPED BY THE ACTIVITY PSYCHOTHERAPY GROUPS

The cases of Mrs. P. and Mrs. A. show the validity of the activity group psychotherapy approach in relieving the emotional problems of elderly individuals. Their cases also demonstrate the development of leadership skills by the group members.

Mrs. P. was referred to the Outlook Clinic in 1979 by a local social worker. Her chief complaints at the time of admission to the clinic were (1) social isolation, (2) conflicts with her stepgrandson, (3) temper outbursts, and (4) difficulty adjusting to her chronic illness (Waller's disease).

Mrs. P. was a seventy-five-year-old white widow living in subsidized housing with her eighteen-year-old black stepgrandson. An only child, she had lost her middle-class Irish Catholic parents early in life. In addition, a grandparent had tricked her out of her inheritance. Attending parochial schools and completing two years of college, she then worked at a variety of jobs, including that of paymaster of a large company. She married a black man and became stepmother to his children. Her husband had died eight years prior to her admission, and for seven years prior to admission she had lived with and raised her stepgrandson.

Isolated and depressed, Mrs. P. described her life: "I spend most of my time watching TV and I rarely go out of my home to see friends." During her first two years at the clinic, she received individual and group counseling. She liked the groups because they involved her in activities (arts and crafts and painting), as well as in discussions of problems. She said she could participate in the groups, despite being shy, because she knew one of the leaders from the community. She liked the leader of the other group because she was dynamic: "She was the type of person who could get you interested in doing something new." Mrs. P. recalls she had always been afraid to draw, but with this leader's encouragement she was able to execute a variety of creative pieces. The art also provided a vehicle for her to discuss life problems. In individual therapy she recognized her need to set firmer limits on her grandson. She also came to realize the connection between her ambivalent feelings toward him and her unresolved feelings about her own childhood. As she started to resolve these feelings, her temper outbursts decreased.

Mrs. P.'s remarkable development from a dependent client to a peer leader occurred in the arts and crafts group and warrants a detailed description. I first met Mrs. P. when I started as a consultant to the arts and crafts group in 1980. At that time the client was observed to be dependent, passive, and negativistic. She was very reluctant to start her projects, complaining that she was incapable. She related primarily to the group leaders and required much individual attention. Rarely did she relate to the other members of the group. Her primary topics of conversation were her personal concerns, such as her conflicts with her grandson and concern over her chronic illness. The staff constantly encouraged interaction, and gradually she related more openly with the other group members. Eventually she became good friends with another group member, Mrs. A.

Mrs. A., a sixty-three-year-old widow, was the daughter of Lithuanian immigrants. Born and raised in Boston, she lives alone and has limited contact with her family. She worked on assembly lines during World War II, like "Rosie the riveter," and once sustained multiple injuries when she fell down a factory elevator shaft. This accident occurred on a night she was substituting for her mother. Although she worked for a number of years later as a waitress, the injuries impaired her mobility and forced her to retire a few years ago. Since her retirement, Mrs. A. has been active in a variety of community affairs, such as helping to organize an acting group and serving as a board member of the local health clinic.

At first Mrs. P. was quite dependent on her new friend. Mrs. A. was the strong, helpful member in the relationship, while Mrs. P. frequently put herself down and expressed neediness.

In the fall of 1981 the two agreed to become assistants to the group leaders. During the next six months Mrs. A. was an active helper in the group, while Mrs. P. suffered an exacerbation of her medical condition and in addition developed arthritis. As a result, Mrs. P. participated inconsistently during this period.

In the spring of 1982 my coleader announced that she needed to take a five-week leave of absence. The group decided that during that time Mrs. A. would assist me as leader. Before long, however, Mrs. A.'s old injuries flared up and Mrs. P. had to take over as assistant leader. In the process, Mrs. P. underwent a remarkable transformation in behavior and personality. She became motivated to help other members in the group and Mrs. A. outside of it. She reminded members when the next meeting was to occur. She thought up appropriate projects for each member and gently encouraged them to try new tasks. She also was sensitive to mood changes in the members and helped them to discuss their problems.

Mrs. A. recovered and returned to the group. There she assisted Mrs. P., a role in which she seemed most comfortable. The two complemented each other excellently, both inside and outside the group. Mrs. A. was very practical and had excellent dexterity, but tended to avoid discussing feelings. Mrs. P. had developed an excellent social and emotional sensitivity, but lacked some practical and crafts skills. Together they continued to assist in leading the group until the clinic closed in 1983.

POLICY ISSUES

Savings Produced by the Outlook Clinic

During the five years of clinic operation less than 10 percent of the clients were transferred to chronic-care facilities. Furthermore, there were numerous examples of clients whose use of medical emergency rooms and acute care hospitals dramatically decreased during their participation in the Outlook groups.

This experience corresponds with other workers who have shown that psychotherapy reduces utilization of medical facilities (Mumford, Schlesinger, Glass, Patrick, and Cuerdon, 1984). Given the high cost of medical services (up to five hundred dollars per person per day) and the low cost of our program (five hundred dollars per person per year), it is clear that our activity psychotherapy groups were economical as well as humane.

Influence of Funding Sources on the
Operation of the Psychotherapy Groups

Under the AOA grant period. During this period group leaders were selected primarily according to their ability to blend interpersonal and activity skills. Since this combination is rarely taught in more formal programs, it was necessary to seek leaders among the less traditional training programs such as expressive therapy. Furthermore, the clients were not billed for the services, so they did not have to identify themselves as clients as much as group members.

Under Medicare and Medicaid funding. In 1981, at the recommendation of AOA, we shifted our funding source to Medicare and Medicaid. This shift in funding raised a variety of policy issues, such as staffing pattern, patient stigma, and model of treatment. With regard to staffing, Medicare requires that a psychiatrist be present to conduct each therapy session. Not only is this highly expensive, it is also inappropriate: psychiatric training does not include activity group psychotherapy.

Medicare funding also means that the group members are defined as psychiatric patients; they are sent a receipt saying they received psychiatric services. For a majority of the elderly, being a psychiatric patient means you are crazy. The practitioner is thus confronted with the dilemma of how adequately to inform group members of the nature of the service without scaring them away.

Medicare funding also means that services must conform with the standards of the necessity for treatment and the appropriateness of the mode of treatment as established by local peer review organizations. This creates a further barrier to any psychiatrist attempting to conduct an activity psychotherapy group of the type described here.

CONCLUSION

Activity group psychotherapy is an effective mode of treating the emotional and social needs of the inner-city elderly. These groups reduce the isolation and loneliness seen in this population. They provide the elderly a respectful and acceptable form of discussing the numerous emotional issues that might otherwise cause mental disorders. These groups are highly cost-effective, as they reduce institutionalization and the utilization of costly medical services. They are also humane, as they assist the elderly in living more of their last years in a dignified setting. Let us hope more funding will become available for these groups.

REFERENCES

Birren, J. E., & Sloane, R. B., Eds. (1980), *Handbook of Mental Health and Aging*. Englewood Cliffs, N.J.: Prentice-Hall.

Blackman, D. K., Howe, M., & Pinkston, E. M. (1976), Increasing participation and social interaction in institutionalized elderly. *Gerontologist*, 16:69–76.

Butler, R. N., & Lewis, M. I. (1982), *Aging and Mental Health: Psychosocial Approaches*. St. Louis: Mosby.

Leiff, J. (1984), *Your Parent's Keeper: A Handbook of Psychiatric Care for the Elderly*. Cambridge, Mass.: Ballinger.

Mumford, E., Schlesinger, H. J., Glass, G. V., Patrick, C., & Cuerdon, T. (1984), A new look at evidence about reduced cost of medical utilization following mental health treatment. *Amer. J. Psychiat.*, 141:1145–1158.

Reichenfield, H. F., Csapo, K. G., Carriere, L., & Gardner, R. C. (1973), Evaluating the effect of activity programs on a geriatric ward. *Gerontologist*, 13:305–310.

9

Groups for Widowed and Lonely Older Persons

JEANETTE HAINER, A.C.S.W.

The condition of widowhood is accompanied by many complex transitions. At first there are several stages of grief and mourning around the death of a spouse (Kubler-Ross, 1969; Silverman, 1981). The successful completion of this initial task yields to confronting the strangeness, isolation, and loneliness of widowhood. Adaptation to widowhood takes place in the last stage of the process with the redefinition of one's role, an acceptance of one's changed status, and a new sense of oneself. At each of the stages the stress of the transition can be eased by group interventions.

Widowhood has a prominent role in our society, as a statistical portrait of the American widow shows: the average age of widowhood is fifty-six; 68 percent of all women are widows at age seventy-five; the average woman can expect ten years of widowhood. There are five widows to every widower. It is estimated that 40 percent of all older widows live on or below the poverty level and that three-fifths of all widows live alone or with nonrelatives (Porcino, 1983). Most women in this vulnerable social group have not planned ahead for independence in their later years. When a woman's sense of self is linked primarily to her role as wife, the loss of the attachment will be damaging to her very identity (Silverman, 1981). Widowhood is a major life change and requires more adjustment than almost any other life event (Porcino, 1983).

In addition to attending to legal and financial matters and to the details of daily life, widowed persons are simultaneously grieving the loss of a mate with whom they have spent, for better or for worse, most of their adult lives. It is generally accepted that the period of mourning lasts between three months and a year (Weiner and Teresi,

1983). The pain of grief is a normal reaction to the stress caused by loss (Lindemann, 1944). Physical symptoms and feelings experienced during this period, though sometimes extreme, may be psychologically appropriate and even healthy (Toth and Toth, 1980; Silverman, 1981).

The loss of a spouse reveals the strengths and vulnerabilities of the remaining partner. That there are extreme reactions to the stress factor in an already vulnerable spouse is illustrated by the fact that the suicide rate after widowhood is exceeded only by the rate after divorce and separation, which is about two and a half times greater than that for the general population (Verwoerdt, 1979). Informal and formal group support can intervene at this time.

The grief process is eased when one is surrounded by the comfort and closeness of loved ones. These informal support systems can help a widow or widower through the normal grief process. When relatives, friends, and others do not understand the grief process—when they treat the widowed person as "sick" or incapable of making decisions—they are undermining attempts by the grieving person to put his or her life back in order. The people to whom one traditionally may be expected to turn at a time of loss may be unavailable when needed.

Lopata (1979a, 1979b), in her study of resources and support systems of widows in metropolitan Chicago, found a dramatic failure of the helping professions—priests, ministers, rabbis, and physicians—to support the wife either during her husband's illness or in the life-rebuilding stage. By contrast, formal group interventions are structured to focus on the widowed person's needs.

At Montefiore Medical Center in New York City a study of widows and widowers with major problems revealed that the continuous lack of the "tranquilizing influence" of human companionship leaves this group more susceptible to physical and emotional illness. Those widows and widowers who received several months of supportive psychotherapy to aid them through the grief process were less likely to require medical treatment or medication than those who did not receive the psychotherapy (Porcino, 1983).

At Sisters of Charity Hospital in Buffalo, New York, André and Susan Toth conducted six-session groups with twelve women who were widowed no less than six months and no more than fourteen. By the end of the first session these women had become a cohesive group with a strong bond. By the sixth session one of the group members stated: "After listening to each lady tell her sad story, it suddenly became clear that I wasn't alone anymore. I found a place I belonged. I am a widow and so are all the other ladies" (Toth and Toth, 1980, p. 63). These conclusions highlight the need for bereavement clinics and support groups.

Groups for widowed persons can be conducted in a variety of settings outside the traditional mental health agency. Possible locations are housing units, senior centers, extended care facilities, and day care centers (Burnside, 1978), as well as in Y's and adult and continuing education institutions.

We are seeing the growth of mutual aid and self-help groups in a variety of settings. Being surrounded by others who understand—who have been through or are going through a common experience —provides emotional support that helps mitigate feelings of isolation and loneliness. Additionally, this supportive environment provides an opportunity to receive information and to learn creative ways of adapting to a new role, thereby reducing stress and reinforcing one's ego strength. Mutual help networks are encouraged within and without a professional setting. With the increasing size of the elderly population and the limitations on professional services available, the mutual help philosophy can reverse the loss of social role which older people experience (Ehrlich, 1979).

Widowed persons who have not gone through the normal grief process often manifest symptoms and behavior that lead others to direct them to seek professional help or to socialization groups where they can be with others of similar age and status. Referrals may come from family members, the family physician, a psychiatrist, a social worker in a social agency, a neighbor, or a friend. Often it is an adult child who makes the referral. This may be both out of concern for the remaining parent's well-being and for his or her own fears of obligation to the remaining parent. More frequently, the widowed person is self-referred, recognizing a need to be with others. Inclusion in a bereavement group is short-term and may either precede participation in a more diverse group or be concurrent with it.

There appear to be different reactions for men and women. A widowed man has a less difficult time being accepted and included. His social position is more secure (Weiner and Teresi, 1983). On the other hand, a widow, who is often felt to be a burden, tends to be avoided. As a result she is expected to keep a "stiff upper lip" and not display her grief (Toth and Toth, 1980).

Widowers are less likely to seek help when needed (Lopata, 1979a, 1979b). As director of a large social, recreational, and cultural program for older adults, it is my experience that although men are more apt to be self-referred at the time of retirement, they are less likely to seek the group on their own initiative at the time of widowhood. Usually they will be directed by a child, a female friend, or a neighbor.

Lopata finds that widowers are still uncomfortable in the home and are reluctant to plan social activities. There is research that points to the fact that men who are widowed prove to be more vulnerable to life's adversities and have lower "well-being" than widowed women. This may be related to the loss of care previously provided by the wife, who was the nurturing spouse (Grove, 1973). It is found that as a result widowed men participate less in social activities and are more isolated than are women. Moreover, men, who often have to assume housekeeping functions, may be uncomfortable in this new role, which they may consider demeaning, whereas widowhood often allows women to expand their responsibilities and decision making (Arens, 1982–1983). Coping capacity may be greater for women, who are often younger than men when they are widowed and who also, because of the greater number of widowed women, have more opportunity to prepare themselves for widowhood.

Recently, through the National Self-Help Clearinghouse, a self-help support group for widowers was started and, in New York City, at the Graduate School and University Center of City University, is holding ongoing socialization and lecture groups.

There is no cure for loneliness but people. The quality of the emotional support provided by one's social network greatly determines the way an individual will respond to a new stage of life (Silverman, 1981).

When the grief work is finished, the widowed person is ready to begin to investigate new relationships. One cannot, however, establish satisfactory relationships until one has adjusted to the grief and emerged as a person who has something to offer others (Peterson, n.d.).

Primary sources for a sense of well-being for both men and women are good health, participation in recreational activities, and socializing with friends (Arens, 1982–1983). No longer having the social context of marriage as a source of well-being, the lonely person needs a protective environment that will provide an opportunity to develop interpersonal connections and share common beliefs and values.

Often such an environment may be experienced as a "second home" or may function as an extended family. Group services for older persons provide this opportunity. To view it from another perspective, lonely people can experience more enjoyment from their own home by having another source readily available for stimulation. Equally, when the burden of a lonely person's feelings are not placed primarily on family members, more satisfying family relationships can occur. When widowed persons are not overdependent on adult children and family for their social needs; when they have age, interest, and situationally appropriate sources to meet these needs independently, the family can then be available to fulfill their needs for closeness and affiliation. This will serve to enrich the lonely person's life. It will also enhance the health of the family system.

Loss does not occur to the widowed person alone; an entire system is impacted. Group services that support continued independence further the opportunity for growth and development for an older person; in fostering positive adaptation and a positive role image, they help dispel fears of role reversal and thus prevent disturbances in the larger family.

When parents, just as their children before them, allow themselves to remain dependent and to allow others to determine their lives in important ways, they can expect to feel angry, bitter, and disappointed. Conversely, parents who remain independent, assertive, and in charge of their lives may feel guilty for "deserting" their children (Weiner, 1983).

Widowhood continues to be complex as necessary adjustments are made to the many shifts in the family and social systems. With the loss of a spouse there is no longer a partner nor the likelihood of a parent to turn to for consolation. Adult children, too, experience loss. The loss of a parent and spouse marks a very delicate time in the family, and shifts of dependency may occur. An environment shared with others who are experiencing similar feelings and interactions allows for support and understanding, and often acts as a stabilizer in helping one focus on healthy priorities. The opportunity is available to talk about changing roles, to laugh together about things older people know that younger people don't. Sharing with one's peers serves to continue a sense of mastery, builds self-esteem, and encourages separateness and differentiation. When there is no association with a group, role boundaries may become blurred at times of vulnerability, thereby weakening the sense of self.

Widowhood is both an ending and a new beginning. Eleanor Kantor used to come with her husband to the senior center for the weekly folk dance class. Suddenly she found herself a widow. Her comments to me over time indicated how she used the group to work through her feelings and for support. In the earlier stages of her loss she would say, "I've seen others survive, so I know I will too." As time progressed, she participated in additional activities and came to the center more frequently. With each new endeavor she became critical and expressed feelings of deprivation. However, she continued to increase her involvement. She reported that it was too difficult for her to manage some tax and financial matters, which her husband had always handled. She investigated and found a way to free herself from the troublesome details. Her initial self-centeredness, necessary to the grief and healing process, has yielded to a caring of self and an ability to take from and share with others. Now, as she observes others in those "initial" stages, she comments, "They'll learn."

Porcino (1983) cites a vignette that further illustrates the ability for growth and change:

At age 57 my husband died suddenly of cardiac arrest. For the first year I walked the shopping malls rather than come home to an empty house. It soon became apparent that I was a fifth wheel in our "coupled" society, which made me feel uncomfortable enough to start declining invitations. However, despite all of this, life without my husband has had some positives. I've always loved to travel, but my husband didn't. In these five years I've traveled to Hawaii, camped my way across the country with my two adult children, and toured Italy. I also have the freedom to take some really interesting adult education courses. I'm less materialistic now, and I have a new appreciation of life and greater clarity about what is important. [p. 42]

Being old is not synonymous with being inflexible. Myths about lack of productivity, disengagement, and senility perpetuate injustices and prejudice against older people. This can be explained in part by lack of knowledge and insufficient contact with a wide variety of older people (Butler, 1975). A sense of personal growth throughout the course of life is essential. Limiting one's self-development and self-expression is to run the risk of becoming frozen into a rigid role (Butler, 1970). The group environment can be a safe harbor for mitigating these stereotypes and myths.

Companionship and group involvement, while helping to limit lonely feelings, may not alleviate them. Intimacy, the warmth and closeness of a physical relationship, and sex are not easily available when the ratio of men to women is one to five. Again, this is less a problem for men, who are sought after and who tend to have to do little in the way of initiation, although their less-developed social skills may make for a more difficult transition.

It is predicted that people who have been sexually active throughout life will be desirous of sexual activity in later years (Butler and Lewis, 1977). Group activities can be developed to provide opportunity for physical touch. A group atmosphere can encourage the enjoyment of intimacy. There may even be love matches within the group. Unfortunately, however, society has little sympathy for sex among older people, and especially among single seniors. Solutions are not readily available or acceptable (Peterson and Payne, 1975). However, this does not diminish the value of the contributions that groups can make to older, lonely, widowed persons.

REFERENCES

Arens, D. A. (1982–1983), Widowhood and well-being: An examination of sex differences within a causal model. *Internat. J. Aging and Human Devel.*, 15:27–40.

Burnside, I. M. (1978), *Working with the Elderly: Group Process and Techniques.* North Scituate, Mass.: Duxbury Press.

Butler, R. N. (1970), Looking forward to what? *Amer. Behav. Scientist*, 14 (Sept.):121–128.

——— (1975), *Why Survive?* New York: Harper & Row.

——— Lewis, M. I. (1977), *Sex After Sixty.* New York: Harper & Row.

Ehrlich, P. (1979), Service delivery for the community elderly: The mutual help model. *J. Gerontol. Social Work*, 2:125–135.

Grove, W. R. (1973), Sex, marital status and morality. *Amer. J. Sociol.*, 79:45–67.

Kubler-Ross, E. (1969), *On Death and Dying.* New York: Macmillan.

Lindemann, E. (1944), The symptomatology and management of acute grief. *Amer. J. Psychiat.*, 101:141–149.

Lopata, H. (1979a), Widows and widowers. In: *The Age of Aging: A Reader in Social Gerontology*, ed. A. Monk. Buffalo: Prometheus, pp. 214–222.

——— (1979b), *Women and Widows.* New York: Elsevier.

Peterson, J. A. (n.d.), *On Being Alone.* NRTA-AARP-AIM Guide for Widowed Persons. 1909 K Street N.W., Washington, D.C. 20049.

——— Payne, B. (1975), *Love in the Later Years.* New York: Association Press.

Porcino, J. (1983), *Growing Older, Getting Better.* Reading, Mass.: Addison-Wesley.

Silverman, P. R. (1981), *Helping Women Cope with Grief.* Beverly Hills: Sage.

Toth, A., & Toth, S. (1980), Group work with widows. *Social Work*, 25:63–65.

Verwoerdt, A. (1976), *Clinical Geropsychiatry*. Baltimore: Williams & Wilkins.
Weiner, M. B., & Teresi, J., with Streich, C. (1983), *Old People Are a Burden, but Not My Parents*. Englewood Cliffs, N.J.: Prentice-Hall.

10

Group Intervention for Alcohol-Related Problems among the Elderly and Their Families

ELOISE RATHBONE-McCUAN, Ph.D., M.S.W.

Much of the empirical knowledge we have available about alcoholism and aging has been produced in the past decade (Barnes, 1982). At present there are considerable discrepancies in the data describing the prevalence of drinking and the extent of alcohol-related problems in the aging population. The different rates of geriatric alcoholism reported can be partly explained by the variety of methodological approaches used in measuring alcohol use and abuse, and by the fact that some samples are drawn from the general population, others from institutional/clinical settings. Counte, Salloway, and Christman (1982) categorized most of the research on alcoholism and aging as either epidemiological or phenomenological. Both types of research have advanced the field but have also produced many unanswered questions about treatment. The search for causal theories in epidemiological work has not suggested many approaches to the prevention of alcoholism in later life. Phenomenological approaches have typically treated alcoholism as a unidimensional syndrome and are not especially helpful in explaining the clinical variations in the psychosocial dynamics of older alcoholics.

One point of agreement emerging from comprehensive reviews of data is that a bilateral theory of aging and alcoholism is an acceptable preliminary framework for research and intervention. Wood (1982) refers to the two broad groups of elderly alcoholics as early-onset and late-onset types. Zimberg (1982) clusters the alcoholic elderly into the same clinical types and suggests that personality dynamics, crisis problems, and treatment approaches should differ for the two groups. Early-onset elderly alcoholics have been alcoholic earlier in their life. Sometimes these are individuals who have aged with their alcoholism which already in early midlife was a chronic condition. For the late-onset second type, alcohol abuse, prompted by social, psychological, and physical losses, becomes problematic at a later stage of development. Here alcohol abuse may be a coping mechanism seriously compounding other mental health problems.

Current research is helping to debunk a number of myths concerning alcoholism among the elderly. Major points confirmed include (1) the continued biochemical variability of the impact of alcohol consumption across the span; (2) the importance of bringing alcoholism research into the mainstream of biomedical and psychosocial research in aging; (3) the presence of heavy drinking among cohorts of elderly women; (4) a general tendency for alcohol consumption to decline among the elderly; (5) increased drug reaction risks associated with combined and unmonitored use of alcohol and prescribed drugs; (6) isolation as both cause and consequence of alcoholism; (7) favorable prognosis for recovery among elderly alcoholics in treatment; (8) patterns and dynamics of alcoholism that do not produce a homogeneous condition among elderly drinkers; and (9) the fact that limited amounts of alcohol are not necessarily harmful to most older people.

Some of the important clinical symptoms of alcohol consumption and reaction to intoxication have been investigated. While more controlled studies are needed to explain the complex relationship between alcohol and biochemical and physical functions of the aged, clinical observations of elderly persons going through periods and phases of detoxification are significant. Whanger and Meyers (1984) suggest that a diagnosis of intoxication of an elderly individual is appropriate when there is a recent history of alcohol intake with at least one sign of physiological change, such as slurred speech, incoordination, or face flushing, and at least one psychological change, such as mood change, irritability, talkativeness, or impaired thought. Psychological and physical change are evident also during periods of alcohol withdrawal, which may occasion major health risks for some elderly people.

In the lives of most elderly alcoholics and problem drinkers there may be a combination of mental health issues that entangle themselves in the alcohol abuse. Individuals in both groups can experience be-

reavement, depression, physical illness, fear of death, and other traumas and stresses of aging. While general treatment guidelines suggest
that early-onset, chronic alcoholics need behavior therapy or behavior
modification while late-onset subjects require psychosocial treatment,
the picture is not entirely clear. The practitioner seeking definitive
answers about the dynamics of aging and alcoholism must be aware
that both gerontology and geriatric research are in their infancy, and
that debates continue as to the nature and treatment of alcoholism.
For now, the best the practitioner can do is to view the treatment of
alcohol problems among the elderly from a social health approach
(Rathbone-McCuan, 1982).

DEVELOPING A COMPREHENSIVE APPROACH
TO SERVICE DELIVERY

One of the most comprehensive efforts to design a treatment
system to respond to the needs of older alcoholics was launched in
1977 by the governor of Michigan. A Citizen Task Force on Seniors
and Substance Abuse was appointed which by 1981 had taken several
key steps toward developing a service and outreach strategy. The first
problem facing the task force was an absence of information about
the problems of drug misuse and alcoholism. Analyses of survey data
on 1,750 elders showed the parameters of problem drinking in the
community population. When the ages of persons in substance abuse
treatment centers were matched with problem prevalence estimates,
one conclusion was clear: older people were not being treated in
formal substance abuse programs in numbers proportionate to the
prevalence of the problem among them.

A comprehensive goal of upgrading service throughout the state
could be realized only through the involvement of two state agencies
that guide service planning—the aging service network and substance
abuse services. Under a mutual agreement prompted by the task force,
the Michigan Office of Services to the Aging and the Michigan Office
of Substance Abuse Services began a series of cosponsored demonstration projects. The original goals of the demonstration projects
were to design and apply models of intervention into alcohol and
other substance abuse problems of the elderly. The first problem to
be tackled was drug misuse among the elderly. It was selected first
because it was conceived accurately to be a more broad-based public
health problem.

In subsequent years, the project developed a dual focus on alcoholism and drug misuse. Rathbone-McCuan, Peltz, and Resch (1983) analyzed why this project was successful despite its multi-site and interagency complexities. From a social service planning perspective, it was successful because it attempted to introduce cooperation among aging and alcoholic source administrators as a means of commiting resources from both systems to serve older alcoholics. An organization planning approach that moves resources from the top down to the level of direct treatment and care seems necessary. Practitioners cannot effectively treat the elderly alcoholic without a system of care.

A comprehensive adult care continuum of alcoholism treatment services combines inpatient and outpatient services that are systematically organized. Some of the additional resources needed by older alcoholics include access to long-term care settings where attention is given to alcoholism problems, social and leisure opportunities that replace the role of job activities for younger people, and special case management supports.

In addition to these formal services, older alcoholics profit from access and participation in AA groups. Fortunately, most alcoholism treatment settings maintain a formal link with community-based AA (Kurtz, 1984). In Michigan and throughout the country, AA groups are a core part of treatment. By contrast, services for the aged tend to have no automatic link with sources of treatment for alcoholics. Many people working in senior citizen programs have no knowledge about alcoholism, how to identify alcoholism problems among the elderly, or where to refer people for help. Several of the most important aspects of the Michigan project were the links established between the aging and alcoholism services and educating service providers about alcoholism in later life.

The process of designing a treatment system for older alcoholics may not require designing new service resources. On the other hand, funds for professional training are needed to give practitioners the knowledge and skills to work with late-life alcoholism. While a variety of treatment approaches were used in the Michigan service demonstration sites, group-based therapy was the primary service for most clients.

GROUP THERAPY AS A TREATMENT MODALITY

Elderly alcoholics in all treatment situations should be encouraged or required to participate in group intervention. Alcoholics

Anonymous first demonstrated the effectiveness of groups for help-ing alcoholics (Fox, 1962). Currently many alcoholism treatment set-tings indicate groups as the treatment of choice due to its continued effectiveness (Cohen and Spinner, 1982). The rationale for applying group interventions has also been demonstrated in clinical practice with the elderly (Lowy, 1979, 1982).

Group interventions can have numerous treatment objectives and be combined with other services. Some of the more common goals of group treatment applied to elderly alcoholics include (1) education about the disease of alcoholism, (2) confrontation of various common defense mechanisms, (3) exploration of nonalcoholic lifestyle options, and (4) socialization possibilities to avoid isolation. The most fre-quently encouraged form of group involvement is AA. Participation is a readily available option to help an elderly person deal with al-coholism. These groups provide personalized outreach, involve no money, and provide much ongoing personal support and socializa-tion. The exact number of American elderly active in AA remains undocumented, but their numbers are significant. Extensive use should be made of AA groups, but other types of group intervention directed by professionals are also essential.

No single theory of group treatment for older alcoholics has been widely accepted. An integrative framework that combines knowledge of clinical geriatric and group work and alcoholism group treatment is a reasonable departure point for determining how to plan and implement group intervention. Lowy (1982), the leading specialist in clinical group practice with the elderly, identified a range of purposes for using group work with the impaired elderly. These purposes fit directly into the treatment themes appropriate for older alcoholics. Elderly alcoholics require rehabilitation in order to maintain sobriety and/or recover from alcohol-related dysfunction. Their lives require social and emotional enhancement to lessen depression and isolation. Many need to learn new health behaviors, values, and life styles.

While the number of group approaches to the treatment of adult alcoholics seems almost endless, certain components are very com-mon. Phased treatment (Cohen and Spinner, 1982) involves orien-tation, alcohol education, attention to individualized issues, exploration of sobriety as a life style, and active group therapy. This progression can be applied in geriatric treatment.

How the active phase of group therapy is conducted depends on specific goals. Glassman and Wright (1983) propose three general sets of goals that seem to encompass much of group treatment. "Therapy-in-the-group" represents a format where the interaction is primarily between therapists and individual group members. Interaction between the individual group member and the therapist is primary; interaction among group members secondary. This pattern of group process is used in geriatric group work because some elderly group members prefer to relate more directly to the therapist than to peers. Some passive, shy, or functionally impaired members prefer to be observers. Experience suggests that highly frail or cognitively impaired elderly persons may benefit from this type of group experience because constant, intense, and demanding interaction among members may be beyond their functional capacity. Using a group format that matches the interactional capabilities of the elderly members is a key to effectiveness.

"Therapy-in-the-group" is often very useful. Sometimes the measure of therapeutic or personal value of group participation simply means that elderly people can spend time in a group context and feel enhanced by being in the presence of their peers and a trusted therapist. Individualized listening and observing can be a highly stimulating and profitable way for older people to receive help. The subjective value of this style of participation is reflected in the statements of elderly group members: "I learn a lot by hearing others talk and I can think about my troubles"; "It is good to be there because I feel welcome even though I don't say much"; "If I want to get well it means I have to learn how to listen to what others did to get well, not talk about what I haven't done."

"Therapy-with-the-group" is an alternative structure applied by some therapists. Group interaction is considered central. Interpersonal issues are the focal point of sessions, with priority given to the common problems that confront all members. Unlike the first approach, here *process* is considered the most powerful therapeutic force. Experimental sharing among alcoholics and the imparting of common and individual insights into alcohol problems is an accepted form of treatment. A similar focus on problem solving by the members can be used with the variety of psychological and social problems that elderly persons commonly face, such as the death of a spouse or adaptation to an illness or physical impairment.

A less frequently used approach in alcoholism treatment is one that defines the interactive qualities of the group as primary. "Membership-in-the-group" is considered a central goal and the therapeutic interaction is directed to maintaining the group. Emphasis is on the group's development and continuation. This approach has been used in a wide range of socialization and recreational groups for elderly persons who are isolated and need help in reconstructing a social network after a major loss or transition. The tasks that groups complete are often external to the problems of members' private lives, but significant to the way they live their lives in collective experiences.

Whatever type of group is applied with older alcoholic members, *it is essential that an emphasis on conscious material be maintained.* This principle of group practice is emphasized by Lowy (1982) and has a particular clinical meaning for older alcoholics. Dealing with overcoming alcoholism or any other goal related to recovery must be reality-directed. Much of the group interaction or therapist-member interaction is anxiety provoking and confrontational in a supportive manner. The issues that elderly people face about their alcoholism are immediate and tangible. It is very easy for unconscious material, highly encouraged in traditional group psychoanalysis, to drift away from the key behavioral and cognitive problems of the moment. One question deserving attention is how to balance a concern with past events, the need of group members to participate in reminiscence, with attention to more immediate topics and the dynamics feeding into current problems in mental health.

Dunlop, Skorney, and Hamilton (1982) describe the group treatment approach they instituted as part of the demonstration treatment project funded by the National Institute for Alcoholic Abuse and Alcoholism. The Clark County program in the state of Washington, like the Michigan program described earlier, build much of the intervention into the aftercare phases of treatment. Group treatment provides the primary ingredient of aftercare. The overall structure of the service program calls for a multidisciplinary team and attempts to provide community education about alcoholism among the elderly. The intervention model uses the family system as part of the group structure for the older alcoholic. They suggest that early involvement of the family group is valuable as a motivation for getting the older person into the active alcoholism treatment. They encourage family members to participate in factual confrontation about alcohol-related behaviors.

Dunlop, Skorney, and Hamilton report various treatment gains to the elderly participants including management of social isolation problems and a learning or regaining of social skills. Rathbone-

McCuan and Hashimi (1982) also reported, as a result of participation in long-term group therapy, improvement in conditions promoting isolation. It seems valuable to encourage group participation in all phases of treatment, but special efforts should be made to continue with support in maintaining sobriety.

In the clinical planning process, practitioners need to complete an in-depth assessment of an individual's mental and physical status and capacity to perform in a group situation (Rathbone-McCuan, 1982). It is good for an elderly person to have the opportunity to explore participation in several groups. For some aged, participation in groups of heterogeneous age is particularly stimulating. Others find groups with members of similar age more attractive and relevant; they feel they afford them a more realistic chance to form important interpersonal relationships. The experimental projects in Washington and Michigan offered access to both types. Usually the choice of group composition is unavailable, because many communities do not have age-specific groups for older alcoholics.

Variations in group treatment also appear in relation to the involvement of family-directed intervention in alcoholism treatment. The first phase of family treatment in the 1940s and early 1950s was devoted to study of the alcoholic marriage and spousal interactions; this gave rise to an emphasis on couple counseling as a component of active therapy. By the early 1970s a family system approach was part of standard counseling procedures used in alcoholism intervention (Anderson and Henderson, 1983). Recognition of the value of family involvement with older alcoholics is only now being realized.

Dunlop, Skorney, and Hamilton (1982) report using several family therapy configurations in geriatric treatment. Couples counseling and family meetings provide a means of educating patients about the problems of alcoholism in the spousal dyad and family system, as well as of sharing the frustrations and anxieties attendant on change and problem solving. One of the common goals of family therapy is that of improving communication both within the family system and between the family and the larger environment. The use of group therapy for older families is becoming recognized as highly valuable in the management of diverse psychological problems and disorders common among the elderly (Eyde and Rich, 1984).

Geriatric alcoholism, like other chronic diseases, may produce high levels of dependency on other family members. When relatives are primary and routine caregivers, managing their caregiving stresses may be easier with group support (Hartford and Parsons, 1982). The dynamics of isolation become central issues that threaten overall family mental health. Such specific issues as the relocation of elderly members who cannot be maintained at home, the management of necessary caregiving functions, long-range planning for family adaptations, and feelings of entrapment converge to increase both the perception and the actual condition of social isolation. Clinicians who staff such groups are assisted if they have an understanding of the impact of aging on the family system.

THE FUTURE OF GROUP TREATMENT OPTIONS

The efficacy of group therapy for alcoholism problems as well as for other geriatric mental health problems is supported by the clinical outcomes of both long- and short-range trials. Group work with alcoholics is an old and trusted approach. The clinical programs reviewed in this chapter have shown that when geriatric alcoholics are placed in group treatment the outcomes are effective. What blocks the development of this approach is the complex problem of obtaining alcoholism services for older people. In a prior analysis of how to accomplish this goal (Rathbone-McCuan, 1982), I suggested that it would be ill advised to create separate care systems for older alcoholics. I recommended that two strategies for expanding and improving sources be implemented. First is to increase the capacity of general adult alcoholism services to reach out and serve the elderly population. This step requires that the many alcoholism counselors with no background in gerontology become acquainted with the aging process and the aspects of aging that are most frequently interactive with alcoholism. The aging service network and long-term care continuum, providing the bulk of the social and health services to the aged, also need to devote attention to the needs of alcoholic elders. Generally, practitioners in geriatric settings know very little about the disease of alcoholism and its dynamics. Education is required if elderly alcoholics are to have the full benefit of geriatric services in the community or in institutional and hospital settings. The therapist interested in this group practice area would be well advised to explore local resources for elderly alcoholics. If some of the described services are not available, it is appropriate to ask community leaders in the fields of alcoholism treatment and gerontology why they are not. Older people with alcohol-related problems and disabilities will be likely to benefit from a variety of group-oriented treatment options. Their recovery can be enhanced if their relatives or intimate caregivers can be reached through educational support and problem-solving groups. Overall, this emerging type of geriatric group practice holds therapeutic promise; the need for it is great and is daily growing greater.

REFERENCES

Anderson, S., & Henderson, D. (1983), Family therapy in treatment of alcoholism. *Social Work in Health Care*, 8:79–94.

Barnes, G. (1982), Pattern of alcohol use and abuse among older persons in a household population. In: *Alcoholism and Aging: Advances in Research*, ed. W. G. Wood & M. Elias. Boca Raton: CRC Press, pp. 3–16.

Cohen, M., & Spinner, A. (1982), A group curriculum for outpatient alcoholism treatment. *Social Work with Groups*, 5:5–14.

Counte, M., Salloway, J., & Christman, L. (1982), Age and sex related drinking patterns in alcoholics. In: *Alcoholism and Aging: Advances in Research*, ed. W. G. Wood & M. Elias. Boca Raton: CRC Press, pp. 17–28.

Dunlop, J., Skorney, B., & Hamilton, J. (1982), Group treatment for elderly alcoholics and their families. *Social Work with Groups*, 5:87–92.

Eyde, D., & Rich, J. (1984), *Psychological Distress in Aging: A Family Management Model*. Rockville, Md.: Aspen.

Fox, R. (1962), Group psychotherapy with alcoholics. *Internat. J. Group Psychother.*, 12:56–63.

Glassman, S., & Wright, T. (1983), In, with and of the group: A perspective on group psychotherapy. *Small Group Behavior*, 1:96–106.

Hartford, M., & Parsons, R. (1982), Use of groups with relatives of dependent older adults. *Social Work with Groups*, 2:77–90.

Kurtz, L., F. (1984), Linking treatment centers with Alcoholics Anonymous. *Social Work in Health Care*, 9:77–84.

Lowy, L. (1979), *Social Work with the Aging*. New York: Harper & Row.

——— (1982), Social group work with vulnerable older persons: A theoretical perspective. *Social Work with Groups*, 2:21–32.

Rathbone-McCuan, E. (1982), Health and social intervention issues with older alcoholics and alcohol abusers. In: *Alcoholism and Aging: Advances in Research*, ed. W. G. Wood & M. Elias. Boca Raton: CRC Press, pp. 29–39.

——— Hashimi, J. (1982), *Isolated Elders: Health and Social Intervention*. Rockville, Md.: Aspen.

——— Peltz, S., & Resch, J. (1983), Aging alcoholic: A summary of the Michigan experiment as a model of outreach and intervention. Paper presented at the Sangamon State University Gerontology Seminar, Springfield, Illinois.

Whanger, A., & Meyers, A. (1984), *Mental Health Assessment and Therapeutic Intervention with Older People*. Rockville, Md.: Aspen.

Wood, W. G. (1982), Theoretical and methodological issues associated with aging research. In: *Alcoholism and Aging: Advances in Research*, ed. W. G. Wood & M. Elias. Boca Raton: CRC Press, pp. 177–188.

Zimberg, S. (1982), Commentary. In: *Alcoholism and Aging: Advances in Research*, ed. W. G. Wood & M. Elias. Boca Raton: CRC Press, pp. 41–43.

Part IV
*Supportive/Rehabilitative
Group Therapy in Institutions*

11

A Geriatric Group in an Acute Care Psychiatric Teaching Hospital: Pride or Prejudice?

RUTH K. GOODMAN, M.S.W.

Group therapy for the elderly is by no means a new phenomenon or untried modality. However, the idea of developing this form in an acute care psychiatric teaching hospital has received scant attention. A review of the literature reveals rich material about groups in out-patient clinics (both medical and psychiatric), senior citizen centers, residential facilities for the chronically frail elderly (both health-related facilities and skilled nursing homes), and in private practice (Spitz, 1984). In many psychiatric hospitals, while short-term inpatient groups do exist, they are not typically geared to the elderly. My experience in implementing such a group over a two-year period (March 1982 to March 1984) has opened up exciting avenues for exploration, and has been rewarding as well as challenging.

IMPETUS

In addition to a natural inclination to combat inherent prejudices and biases toward the elderly with the pride and dignity that should accompany old age, two issues spurred me to form such a group. The first was my professional concern for the care of the geriatric inpatient population in the clinic where I work. This population is small (slightly less than 15 percent of all inpatients are over sixty-five) but increasing. I had variously been exposed, in the course of my clinical work, to repeated comments about how few of the programs were geared specifically to the needs of the older population. Remarks such as "I feel outnumbered here," "there's nothing here for me," or "there's no one to talk to who really understands people my age" were not uncommon. A sixty-five-year-old woman complained of "feeling like a den mother" until she joined the group. In addition, older patients seemed to feel widespread discrimination because of aging, and biases that appeared to effect all aspects of their lives. Not the least of the prejudices were against their own cohorts, and we noted a frequent longing to be dissociated from the "elderly" designation.

The second issue, a very personal one, was the shift in my role in the institution due to an administrative policy requiring me to step down as director of social work at age sixty-five. This naturally forced me to confront the issues of my own diminished function, effectiveness, and self-esteem, and, as never before, my own mortality.

An initial question concerned the real need for such a group, and its therapeutic value. While special activities groups had previously been organized, were still in progress, and had proved effective and necessary, there were no existing "talk" therapy groups designed especially for this population. The educational value of such groups is undeniable, particularly if developed around the themes discussed below (Maxmen, 1984).

OBSTACLES

Initially, despite overt acknowledgment of the need for such a service, and administrative sanction (i.e., a group to cut across all inpatient units), some systems issues emerged suggesting institutional resistance. Problems cited included interference with unit autonomy, scheduling conflicts, and burden on nursing and other staff because of frail and/or confused patients who needed to be escorted to group. In short, the institutional readiness for service delivery to this group was questionable; it was necessary to address each resistance. This required numerous consultations with everyone involved. Typical of group work in such a setting, there was an evident need for flexibility in focus, format, patient age, group composition, location, and time, and for accommodation to other vital therapeutic interventions (including physical and medical tests of all kinds). This took into account the difficulty and constraints in conducting an open-ended group in an acute care hospital where lengths of stay are relatively brief—usually three months at most (Boriello, 1976; Kibel, 1981).

PILOT

A decision was made to pilot the first group on one unit. Although small (twelve beds), this unit had the highest percentage, floorwise, of patients over fifty-five, the age cohort we felt could benefit most from this type of group intervention. Furthermore, these patients seemed naturally to meet in an informal group of their own, one which gravitated to a sitting area outside the nursing station, and so were readily accessible. Space was usually available and the idea had the full endorsement of all unit staff and the ready acceptance of most patients. (One staff member suggested the name "Life Experience Group," as it did not carry the negative connotation of "senior citizen" or "golden age," and this on the whole has been well received.) A member of the nursing staff who took a genuine interest in this age group enthusiastically volunteered to be cotherapist. Unfortunately, because of personal reasons she resigned after almost a year, but the group continued with a student social worker acting as cotherapist to round out the year.

EXPANSION

Originally planned to encompass all units, the second group was started in March 1983 and is still in progress. Some of the same problems persisted (scheduling and therapeutic conflicts, etc.), but we have had continued endorsement by the administration, and interdisciplinary cooperation has been excellent. Importantly for Group II, a senior occupational therapist from the Therapeutic Activities Department, with excellent prior group experience and a particular interest and understanding of the elderly, volunteered her services as cotherapist. The meetings are now held in my office, which, in addition to being spacious enough to accommodate most group sessions, has the advantage of being located on the same floor as Therapeutic Activities, which simplifies coordination of scheduling with patients and staff members.

SELECTION CRITERIA

Selection criteria were fairly flexible for both groups, but there have been slight differences. Whereas it was possible to include very regressed patients in Group I because of their presence on the unit, this was logistically more difficult to manage in Group II. The age range, fifty-five and over, has remained the same. We have not excluded nonverbal or disturbed patients as long as they have self-transport or can be brought to the sessions, and can tolerate the interaction. Initially we were concerned about the difficulty of including patients receiving ECT, but we became increasingly aware that these patients would be able to communicate, despite memory loss and confusion, if seen on days they were not receiving the shock therapy; they have joined us with a great deal of success. This is discussed further on. There are no sex-related, racial, religious, cultural, or ethnic exclusions.

FORMAT

As mentioned previously, because this is an acute care psychiatric inpatient facility, and stays of over three months are the exception rather than the rule, the group is open-ended; the number of sessions per patient is for the most part limited only by length of stay. The group is run twice a week, at a set time, for roughly one hour per session. Scheduling conflicts occasionally arise, but are usually resolved without difficulty.

MODIFICATIONS

Time limitations render impractical many long-cherished shibboleths regarding group process: preinduction, homogeneity, group cohesion derived from close association over long periods of time (Betcher, 1983), and so on. However, constant emphasis on the group as "special" and geared to the needs of those who are growing older has been a unifying force. Although we have constantly refused to accept society's tendency to "rope off" the senior citizen, and have used ourselves to play up strengths and dispel myths, this has occasionally had its problems: one sixty-four-year-old member astutely questioned whether we weren't actually falling into the same societal trap by setting them apart. However, addressing pride, dignity, and accumulated wisdom and experience has proved gratifying (Knopf, 1977). Another source of group cohesion has been the recognition that members' knowledge, deliberation, caution, modesty, and loyalty (Berland and Poggi, 1979) can more than compensate for any deficiencies in the culturally valued areas of agility, energy level, productivity, and sexual attractiveness; this recognition has also helped the members deal with agist prejudice. Additionally, we have emphasized the group as a forum to learn how to create and strengthen opportunities for communication with all age groups.

COTHERAPY

The literature contains many references to the advantages and/or disadvantages of cotherapy in groups, although there is little controlled research about this (Dick, Kessler, and Whiteside, 1980). The decision to conduct the two groups with cotherapists has proved practical for a number of reasons. Group I was coled by a nurse, as mentioned earlier, who volunteered for the task because of her keen interest in the older population. Group II is coled by a senior occupational therapist who volunteered because of a similar interest, and because of excellent experience running activities groups for senior adults. The latter has provided the seasoned coleadership necessary for this undertaking, and has been introduced to and accepted by the group as "an honorary senior citizen." In both instances the cotherapists have been considerably younger than myself, and thus represent a cross-generational interest which, combined with the voluntary nature of the task, is generally and gratefully acknowledged by the group members. This naturally has enabled me to act as a role model for the older population, particularly in relation to our ability to bridge a generation gap. The cotherapy relationship is then a stage for playing this out and for dealing with transference and countertransference issues. The fact that both pairs of leaders were interdisciplinary (social work and nursing, then social work and therapeutic activities), while not at all uncommon in this setting, has provided group members with a strong sense of the commitment of these disciplines to total patient care, and gives us an opportunity to reinforce the contributions from a variety of orientations. There are obvious practical advantages, such as continuity (if one must be absent), a multiplicity of role possibilities, and the ability to provide a refreshing change of style or pace. With our emphasis on caring, on the group as part of total treatment, and on learning experience, group members see us as thoroughly committed to their strengths rather than to their weaknesses. In Group II particularly, it has also enabled us to stress the importance of mental as well as physical efforts. Our professional orientation, grounded in these values and attentive to ego assets, is particularly valuable in a medical setting.

THEMES

The development of key group themes has been absorbing and provocative (Silver, 1950; Wolff, 1962). Repeated orientation of new members to the purpose of the group, necessary because of its open-endedness, has kept us constantly aware of the neediness of this age group, of the hopes, fears, and goals, realistic or not, in lives that tend to become increasingly isolated, lonely, and stultified. Despite the constantly changing membership, there are usually enough "veterans" who have grasped the purpose to explain it to newcomers. As mentioned before, the "specialness" is always emphasized, and mutual support is a popular and sometimes contagious topic.

In line with the name of the group—the Life Experience Group—reminiscences of past experiences and good times are particularly important (Lewis and Butler, 1974; Lesser, Lazarus, Frankel, and Havasu, 1981); they can be used, as reminders of past but not necessarily lost skills, to enhance present means of coping and adapting. Means of communication, both verbal and nonverbal, are often quickly picked up, and this includes double messages. Positive reinforcement is constantly used and no achievement is considered too insignificant to note.

Issues of loneliness, loss of significant others, retirement, death, and bereavement are very common (Butler and Lewis, 1977); the need for mourning these losses is dealt with directly. This frequently leads to discussions of mourning decreased physical functioning, including hearing, sight, and mobility. A frequently discussed fear is of diminished mental functioning, particularly memory loss, and the frustrations and anger caused by helplessness and dependency. This is particularly true if there has been mandatory retirement from useful occupation. (An eighty-nine-year-old man, highly intelligent and fiercely independent most of his life, proved to be a good role model as he discussed a recent serious illness accompanied by depression: "It's taken me all these years to learn how *delicious* it can be to be cared for!") As we constantly emphasize remaining strengths versus weaknesses, what is "do-able" is quickly picked up on and provides an important area for group cohesion. Addressing members' pride, often on an insignificant level, frequently provides the opportunity for self-examination. It also cuts down considerably on expressions of self-pity and worthlessness. Self-acceptance and acknowledgment of age play important roles here and are frequent themes, helping members realistically accept their limitations (Knopf, 1977). We often discuss the rather controversial view of the advantages of growing older; frequently members can see few positives beyond the somewhat questionable Social Security benefits, or reduced fares for public transportation. However, during one session this led to a heated discussion about reactions to being offered a seat on a bus. A sixty-nine-year-old man interpreted such offers as confirmation of his growing feebleness; he felt devalued and insulted, particularly if the offer was made by a woman, and had consistently refused to apply for a senior transportation card. A sixty-four-year-old industrial worker made a point of joining younger people at lunch hour, not willing to be grouped with his peers. However, an eighty-one-year-old woman announced with authority and much dignity, as she pounded the floor with her cane, that she felt she had earned the right to be comfortable! The group then expressed strong positive feelings of being worth this respect, and of increasing self-assurance in asking for it. An example of members caring about each other was movingly illustrated by the insistence of a seventy-five-year-old woman that her roommate, sixty-four years old, withdrawn, apathetic, and depressed, accompany her to this group rather "than lie alone in bed all day." The sixty-four-year-old was at first annoyed at the older woman's insistence, but in the group both realized that the incident was a sign of caring.

Since the majority of our members are admitted for depression, this becomes a frequent theme. The fact that most of the patients improve and can also recognize that they have had successful treatment in the past is a source of benefit. The sense of improvement is usually remarked by others before it is felt by the individual, but frequently has a positive and profound effect on the depressed patient; it is here we can usually introduce the fact that the hospitalization is only a small fraction of total life experience and can be used as a means of learning about oneself. Depression as the result of a combination of biological or chemical imbalances as well as psychosocial stressors is eagerly discussed, and the educational potential of these discussions often mitigates the negative assumption that depression is due to the aging process alone.

The idea of intergenerational gaps is another frequent topic, and makes for lively discussion of stereotypical attitudes going both ways. The realization that older people can make their lives interesting to younger generations provides the former a sense of the continuity of life. The meaning of "roots," of taking an historical perspective, takes on a new and poignant significance for many. Two members in their

sixties, resentfully agreeing that "young people don't want to be both-
ered with us," were astonished when a seventy-year-old woman spoke
of her granddaughter's fascination with her long-ago immigration to
this country from France, and with the customs and traditions she
had brought with her. This reinforced our emphasis on the group as
a means of learning how to relate to all ages, rather than seeing oneself
as "roped off."

The idea of sharing private thoughts and feelings with others,
particularly in a group setting, is ego-alien and quite repugnant to
many group members, depending on age and cultural orientation. A
seventy-two-year-old woman deplored the current fashion among
younger persons of "letting it all hang out," but gradually became
comfortable and open in a setting she felt would guarantee confidentiality and acceptance by her peers. Conversely, we have found
that in a caring, nonjudgmental, and "safe" setting, "talk therapy" can
be productive and therapeutic (Parham, Priddy, McGovern, and Richman, 1982). "I feel I can say what I think" is often expressed and
receives positive feedback.

Sharing of cultural, ethnic, and religious customs is a popular
focus, particularly around holiday times, and leads to the acceptance
of one another's differences and individuality. Often it becomes a
springboard for speaking out against all discrimination, including that
against the elderly. A seventy-four-year-old woman shared with the
group the significance of the Swedish "Little Christmas," brought a
candle to illustrate this, and involved the group in a discussion of the
universality, transcending all ages, religions, and cultures, of cele-
brating the "return" of the sun to the world. As she further stated,
"the way we feel about these things is not dependent on how old we
are."

Two further issues, initially considered too highly charged to deal
with directly, have proven important. The first concerned the meaning to group members of hospitalization in a psychiatric inpatient
setting. Feelings of stigma, shame, and guilt were often layered onto
the natural loss of dignity and pride, making it doubly difficult to
combat bias against aging. Patients have gradually felt free to discuss
the differences between hospitalization for physical causes and for
mental illness. They often skirt the real issues by using such terms as
"emotional troubles" or "nervous disorder"; when we acknowledge
openly that what they fear is "going crazy" or "losing control," they
often become surprisingly verbal and comfortable in discussing such
fears.

The second issue, equally loaded, was the frequent use of ECT as a treatment for severe depression. Initially in Group I, I felt it to be a threatening topic, as discussions were divided between those who had refused it and did not want to know about it, and those under treatment who did not remember it or were reluctant to discuss it. As we dealt with our own feelings about ECT, and since it is so commonly used, we have been able to introduce the topic with regularity. In most sessions more than half the group have had ECT in the past, are in the midst of an ECT course, have just had it prescribed, or have just completed it. While acknowledging the value of individual patient orientation to this modality by other disciplines, the group setting often builds greater confidence. Members frequently bring up the subject themselves, and we have been able to discuss and dispel myths. Fears of permanent brain damage, particularly permanent loss of memory, and the common fear of loss of control are introduced, demystified, and accepted to a surprising degree. Patients awaiting ECT have benefited from observing recovering patients and the positive feedback about the lifting of their depressions; they are thus able to see ECT as another effective means of getting better, along with other modalities in a total treatment program.

In terms of group leadership and style, we tend to be quite active, directive, friendly, supportive, and empathic, while encouraging independence. Behavioral techniques are used along with assertiveness training. While therapeutic taboos discourage physical contact, this writer has always comfortably used a simple handshake at the beginning and end of sessions, which is usually gratefully acknowledged and returned. When this is combined with greeting the patient by name, the results are almost always positive, and a sense of gratitude for being acknowledged is evident. Even regressed patients with physical impairments are generally relieved to find a supporting hand or arm (Goldfarb, 1972).

We find the use of a good deal of humor to be important. Not only is it vital in developing good reality testing, but broadened points of view emerge. If the cotherapists do not always take themselves so seriously, the group is usually quick to follow suit, which we see as a sign of strength. It has also frequently been possible and appropriate to introduce certain "elderly" jokes, which have helped the group develop more positive perspectives. Since many are oriented toward the inevitability of memory loss with age, its frightening aspects are frequently diminished through humor, and memory deficit as the sole property of aging is contradicted. With an emphasis on the "here and now," a more comfortable acceptance of the life cycle evolves, and the role of the elderly survivors is enhanced (Goldfarb, 1972).

IMPLICATIONS FOR CLINICAL CARE

The implications for clinical care in conducting these groups for older persons are various. Many members have stated that the group sessions provide one of the only methods for combating isolation, and for giving them a sense of belonging, importance, acceptance, and improved self-esteem during hospitalization. Remarkably, despite the time-limited nature of participation, many members have learned to recognize some of their maladaptive patterns. They have realized that there are choices to be made, if only in a limited way, and coping mechanisms to be relearned or newly tried. They often find that the quality of their lives can be improved, if only minimally. It is sometimes quite surprising for them to understand by example in a group setting that anger and frustration are normal, not threatening, and can be used positively if appropriately channeled. Particularly among the elderly, people are trained to avoid expressing strong feelings of every sort, and are surprised to find that such expressions are acceptable. Dealing with physical and psychological deficits in themselves or others is also difficult, but group members have shown a remarkable tolerance for this, and have seemed to benefit from seeing themelves in a helping role, or in accepting help from the leaders or other members (Parham et al., 1982).

STATISTICAL DATA

The average age in Group I was 65, with a range of 50–70. Group II had an average of 69 with a range of 55–89. In both groups, not unexpectedly, women far outnumbered men (77 percent in Group I, 71 percent in Group II). Average length of stay in both groups was 1.5 months, with a range of 1 week to 4.5 months. Average number of sessions per patient was 7 in both groups, with a low of 1 and a high of 18 in Group I; there was a low of 1 and a high of 17 in Group II. Average number of patients in Group I was 5, with a low of 2 and a high of 8. Group II showed an average of 7 patients per session, with a low of 2 and a high of 16. Additional data for the two groups is presented in Table 11.1

TABLE 11.1

Payment Methods:	Medicare	Medicaid	Blue Cross	Other
Group I	50%	10%	35%	4%
Group II	49.5%	4.2%	35.7%	10.6%

Ethnic origin:	Caucasian	Black	Hispanic	Other
Group I	95%	5%	–	–
Group II	90.2%	5.5%	1.9%	2.4

Marital Status:	Married	Widowed	Divorced	Separated	Single
Group I	51%	22%	12%	5%	10%
Group II	45%	28%	12%	2%	13%

Religion:	Catholic	Jewish	Protestant	Other	Unknown
Group I	37%	43%	20%	–	–
Group II	30%	40%	11%	12%	7%

Diagnostically, both groups combined showed a high percentage of Axis I depressive disorders (66 percent), with 42 percent Major Depression, recurrent (DSM–III 296.3x), 24 percent Major Depression, Single Episode (DSM–III 296.2x), 8 percent Bipolar Disorder, Depressed (DSM–III 296.5x). Axis II diagnoses were not available at this time.

As for treatment methods, data for Group I showed 74 percent on antidepressants, 36 percent on ECT, 27 percent on lithium, and 6 percent on other psychotropic medication. The treatment methods were often combined. Medications and ECT data is unavailable for Group II.

IMPLICATIONS FOR TEACHING

Although the elderly population in this inpatient hospital is relatively small, it nonetheless is present and its numbers seem to be growing. Given the population "explosion" of elderly far into the next century, are we dealing sufficiently with the problems of this age group to train and teach the various disciplines to handle them (Nininger, Matorin, Goodman, Kaplan, Beverly, and Gibson, 1984)? If working with the older person becomes increasingly a part of the mental health professional's task, are we providing the necessary tools for understanding aging? We believe that insufficient attention is paid to this problem, particularly to dealing with our own feelings and myths about aging and mortality (Butler and Lewis, 1977). We need to teach more about the particular use of psychopharmacology and ECT with the elderly, as well as differential psychopathology. Exposure to these problems in a group setting can be very educational, and a group of older persons can be excellent teachers. As one sixty-six-year-old stated, "I feel like an hourglass whose sand has run out, but in the group I learned that I can turn the glass over." We must learn patience, the ability to question without prejudice, and an acceptance of the realities of living with more and more older persons.

IMPLICATIONS FOR RESEARCH

It seems vital to conduct follow-up studies of the group members, but due to limited resources this has not been feasible. We are interested in the possibility of prolonged benefit from even brief and transitory group experiences. We have had many informal encounters with former patients who remember the group positively and have sought a similar experience after discharge. Feedback is usually that the group has helped raise self-esteem and fostered feelings of "belongingness." Measuring this more objectively would be interesting and informative, especially if we could learn more about carryover to posthospital adjustment.

Since ECT is so widely administered, particularly to older depressed persons in this setting, and was such a prominent theme in our group, it seems vital to study the subjective reactions of these patients to this treatment. We are aware of many studies designed to determine the efficacy and outcome of this particular form of treatment; we would like to see more formal studies geared to the manifold ramifications of such treatment in an acute care psychiatric hospital. We are aware also that there are patients who have returned to this hospital pleading for ECT because it has helped in the past. Similarly, we know of many who dread the very initials. We have noted that the group allows for the expression of deeply felt reactions, pro and con, to such a controversial and little understood form of treatment. These reactions persist with patients and families despite careful orientation by doctors and other staff members. While older patients, given sufficient desperation about their suffering, tend on the whole to be tractable about treatment, a study designed to determine their reactions and the role of this type of group in correcting distortions and dispelling fears would be revealing and worthwhile.

CONCLUSION

The value of group therapy, particularly for the aging, appears to have been well-established. In an acute care psychiatric teaching hospital, it seems vital. While aware that the inpatients described in this chapter participate in and are exposed to a variety of milieu groups and group activities, over two years' experience as a group leader has convinced me of the value of this special endeavor. The cohesion developed in a "talk therapy" group "just for them" has allowed for very broad themes to emerge in a more focused and productive way, particularly in the areas of existing strengths, inherent pride and dignity, and the development of mutual support.

REFERENCES

Berland, D. I., & Poggi, R. (1979), Expressive group psychotherapy with the aging. *Internat. J. Group Psychother.*, 29:87–108.

Betcher, R. W. (1983), The treatment of depression in brief inpatient group psychotherapy. *Internat. J. Group Psychother.*, 33:365–385.

Boriello, J. F. (1976), Group psychotherapy in hospital systems. In: *Group Therapy: An Overview*, ed. L. R. Wolberg & M. L. Aronson. New York: Stratton Intercontinental, pp. 99–108.

Butler, R. N., & Lewis, M. I. (1977), *Aging and Mental Health: Psychosocial Approaches*. St. Louis: Mosby.

Dick, B., Kessler, K., & Whiteside, J. (1980), The developmental framework for cotherapy. *Internat. J. Group Psychother.*, 30:273–285.

Goldfarb, A. I. (1972), Group therapy with the old and the aged. In: *Group Treatment of Mental Illness*, ed. H. I. Kaplan & B. J. Sadock. New York: Dutton, pp. 623–642.

Kibel, H. D. (1981), A conceptual model for short-term inpatient group psychotherapy. *Amer. J. Psychiat.*, 138:74–80.

Knopf, O. (1977), *Successful Aging*. New York: Viking.

Lesser, J., Lazarus, L. W., Frankel, R. A., & Havasu, S. (1981), Reminiscence group therapy with psychotic geriatric inpatients. *Gerontologist*, 21:291–296.

Lewis, M. I., & Butler, R. N. (1974), Life review therapy: Putting memories to work. *Geriatrics*, 29:165–173.

Maxmen, J. S. (1984), Helping patients survive theories: The practice of an educative model. *Internat. J. Group Psychother.*, 34:355–367.

Nininger, J., Matorin, S., Goodman, R., Kaplan, R. D., Beverly, D., & Gibson, C. (1984), A survey of evaluation and treatment of the older patient: Educational oversights? Unpublished manuscript.

Parham, I. A., Priddy, J. M., McGovern, T. V., & Richman, C. M. (1982), Group psychotherapy with the elderly: Problems and prospects. *Psychotherapy: Theory, Research & Practice*, 19:437–443.

Silver, A. (1950), Group psychotherapy with senile psychotic patients. *Geriatrics*, 5:147–150.

Spitz, H. I. (1984), Contemporary trends in group psychotherapy: A literature survey. *Hospital & Community Psychiat.*, 35:132–142.

Wolff, L. (1962), Group psychotherapy with geriatric patients in a psychiatric hospital: 6-year study. *J. Amer. Geriat. Soc.*, 10:1072–1085.

12

Groups for the Terminally Ill Cardiac Patient

WILLIAM WEINER, A.C.S.W.

This chapter describes short-term, open-ended groups for cardiac patients at different stages of their illness, including end state (terminally ill) as well as severe stages. The literature on group work with the terminally ill elderly is in favor of a directive approach with the group leader taking a very active and supportive role. It is held that since many elderly are preoccupied with their many losses, and with anxiety around death and dying, the focus and purpose of the group should be the alleviation of these anxieties (Burnside, 1978). It is held further that insight can be very harmful for this population, and that the major focus should be on creating a supportive environment (Wolf, 1979). Spiegel and Yalom (1978), in "A Support Group for Dying Patients," state that what seems to be a curative factor is the feeling that "we are all in the same boat." This article stresses the importance of helping patients cope with their life-threatening illness rather than giving in to it. The group leader in supportive groups with the elderly should be tuned in to the members' need for help. This can be done by reassurance, guidance, and environmental manipulation if necessary (Weiner, Brok, and Snadowsky, 1978). Lipton and Malter (1971) emphasize the need for a therapeutic milieu aimed at creating changes in the patient by the social worker's opening up of communication between staff and patient. These writers have influenced me in developing the short-term open-ended groups described below.

POPULATION AND GROUP METHOD

All the members in these groups were elderly male veterans (except for one female veteran) in the Bronx Veterans Administration

Hospital. The population for the groups was selected from the cardiac unit. These patients were at various stages of severe cardiac disease.

Since cardiac patients remain in the hospital for a relatively short period (approximately one to four weeks), I proposed an open-ended group which members would attend for however long they stayed; new members were screened for the group as soon as they were admitted to the cardiac unit. The short duration of most patients' stays made it also, of necessity, a time-limited group. It is my feeling that there is a great need for such open-ended groups, especially in general and psychiatric hospitals. Cardiac patients need to focus on their common problems, such as dealing with fears of death and dying, physical limitations, and changes in family systems.

Some writers have questioned whether short-term open-ended groups, with ever changing members, can develop sufficient cohesiveness and group culture to address these foci, which might be more appropriately dealt with in closed groups. For instance, Schopler and Galinsky (1984) raised an interesting question as to whether such groups go through stages of development from preaffiliation to termination. Slavson (1964) who has a psychoanalytic orientation, sees a therapy group as a "closed system." Its very existence depends on this "inbreeding and exclusiveness." Contrary to what other writers believe, it seems to me that these open-ended groups do make gains and do progress over time. This may be due to the ward culture whereby new members, prior to attending group, are filled in as to the purpose of the group; they also see in action the alliances formed between group members. In this way, the group's "beginning" may precede the actual formation of the group—i.e., a form of "group readiness" may be in effect.

PREPARATION FOR THE GROUP

Preparation of Group Members

"Preparation of members will greatly influence the group's fate" (Yalom, 1975). In accordance with this dictum, each new member was screened prior to coming into the group. Group acceptance dictated that hearing and language problems not be present. Sometimes, pressed for time, I would not spend enough time screening and getting to know a new member. This would invariably backfire, in that there would be disruptive behavior and acting out in the group, which would threaten its successful continuation.

The group meetings were held in the day room on Tuesday afternoons from one-thirty to three. The group literature speaks of elderly people being unable to tolerate confinement in a particular place for long periods. I too found, especially with groups smaller than six, that it was desirable to cut the time to one hour. As is usual with open-ended groups, no limit was set as to how many members could attend; most of the time, in fact, there was a shortage of members, attendance ranging from two to ten per session. While Slavson (1964) stated that it takes at least three members to make a group, I found that with even two members present sessions could be very useful.

While attendance was encouraged, it was not mandatory, as might be the case with other hospital groups, such as those run in substance abuse programs. Frequently patients did not want to attend. They may have been lying down after lunch and had to be coaxed into joining the group. Though not actually coerced, they might nevertheless be described as in some sense a captive audience.

Briefing of Staff

One of the most important features of starting and successfully maintaining a group in a hospital setting is to have the sanction of all staff working with the patients. These would include all nursing, physician, and secretarial staff. All personnel should be briefed as to the need and purpose of the group and be reassured that the purpose of the patient group is not to have gripe sessions with complaints about staff and demands for change. Rather, as in the group discussed here, staff should be told that most complaints from members will be seen and handled as expressions of frustration due to their inability to care for themselves as they had in the past. It was pointed out in the present instance that this would be especially true for this mostly elderly and male veteran population, raised in an era when independent functioning was highly valued. When staff are not properly briefed on the group and its function and purpose, disruptions will occur that threaten the group's success and continuity. Since Bronx VA is a teaching hospital, new residents will sometimes insist on taking a patient away from an ongoing group session. This presents a problem in that members feel that the group is less important and has less to offer than services rendered on the medical model. This is no doubt cultural in our society, in which the medical model carries a great deal of prestige and "real help" is thought to come only from medical personnel.

THEMES IN THE GROUP

Depression

The most common problems among the terminally ill elderly are feelings of isolation, helplessness, and hopelessness. This can lead to depression. In order to be helpful it is necessary to be "patiently available and accepting of the realities of the client's situations and feelings" (Herr and Weakland, 1979). "I wish I were dead" should be responded to with "I can certainly understand your feeling that way. I would probably feel about the same in your circumstances." This kind of response helps the elderly patient in that it shows him the reality of his situation. The patient now feels understood, as his reality has been accepted and confirmed. He will now be open to a more positive approach that might help him mobilize himself. The patient's energies should then be directed toward things the patient is able to accomplish despite his illness.

Denial

One of the most important themes in working with the terminally ill elderly is their use of denial. The fatal illness is not only life-threatening but also threatening to the sense of self. By the use of denial "the person is able to preserve his self-esteem" (Weisman, 1972). The wish to deny should therefore be respected, as it can be a very functional coping style. Denial should be addressed only when deleterious to the patient's physical health.

Another important issue related to the elderly patient's use of denial is how it affects all staff working with this population. Weisman states that when a patient uses denial he refutes the reality of the observer. This may be one of the reasons that so many people working with the dying feel it important for patients to come to terms with their life-threatening illness. From my own experience it would seem that what is most helpful is to follow the patient's lead. In other words, if it appears that a patient is using denial, accept this without any attempt at confrontation. Where confrontation has been used, my observation has been that it is probably experienced by the patient as a jarring intrusion; often it results in a further tightening of the defenses.

Weisman describes the differences between terminal cardiac and cancer patients. According to one study, cancer patients were considered by staff to be hopeless, while cardiac patients were viewed as seriously ill with a good chance of recovery. In fact both groups were terminal. Staff were seen as encouraging isolation in cancer patients and supporting their denial. The cardiac patients in this study were found to be much better informed about their illness than were the cancer patients. The latter were seen by staff as more demanding, while the former were better liked.

In my own experience I have found it true that denial is much more prevalent among cancer patients and the staff involved with them than among cardiac patients and their caretakers. Staff members, physicians included, appear much more comfortable speaking euphemistically of a tumor rather than speak the dreaded word: *cancer*. By contrast, a heart condition may be seen as a status symbol in a Protestant work ethic culture. The cardiac condition may show that the male worked hard and long to provide for his family. In group sessions members seemed to reflect this value by stating that they would much rather have their cardiac condition, even if severe, than cancer.

Sometimes patients who are younger than most of the others will say that "each case is very different" when talk centers around their life-threatening illness and how it affects them. The younger patient may then talk about going back to work after a recent heart attack. The group will then come in with how "life is not the same after a heart attack," emphasizing the need to adjust and "slow down." At this point there is usually talk about what one can do and about how physicians never tell patients what they can and should do. One member might point out that it is up to the individual, that everybody is different. Another issue raised frequently by members is that some do too much while others are afraid and do too little.

In one session a member started to say that he does not believe he had a heart attack: friends tell him how good he looks. Other members picked up on this theme, minimizing their cardiac condition by focusing on the other chronic illnesses they suffer from. This I would address by stating that while it is true they have concerns about these other problems, it must be very difficult for them to accept their cardiac condition and the effect it has on them.

Dependency

In most of the sessions medication is an issue and is seen as life-saving. Members for the most part are very knowledgeable about cardiac medications and their side effects. The group for the most part is very positive about medication and usually spends a long time discussing it. While my approach is to be empathic and encouraging of the coping skills evident in such discussions, I would also raise the issue of what it must be like to have to depend on medication. This will bring out feelings of dependency related first to drugs, then to the hospital and the family, usually in that order. Quite often these patients, concerned about their low income, see my primary task as helping them get more money. As this is not the purpose of the group, the overt issue then becomes, what am I doing to help them? Dependency, in this instance, is directed at me. I will point out that I can help them investigate individually their eligibility for whatever additional funds might be available, but that the group itself is meant for the discussion of issues related to the emotional difficulties they might experience in connection with their physical illness. I would then raise the issue that their feelings of not being helped may be related to that illness, to their wish that my omnipotent powers might make them well, and to their disappointment that in fact this is not possible. While expanding this theme, I do make it a point of saying, in relation to their need to see me as an omnipotent healer, that I wish I had that type of power and could use it in their behalf.

Family

Many issues are raised regarding families—spouses, siblings, children—and also friends. Patients often complain of being treated as both invalids and children. They resent being told to "take it easy" or "let me carry that package." Another frequent complaint is that a wife or girlfriend does not want to have sex for fear that "something will happen during the act." (Similarly, they themselves often report the feeling that their heart is a time bomb that may explode at any moment.)

Just as families and friends are often seen as overprotective, so there are cases in which members complain of not being appreciated for how hard they have worked, "killing themselves" to provide for their family. The feeling is that the illness can more readily be accepted by the patient if significant others see it as the result of his attempts to do good and care for others. The fear of not being recognized for who they are appears also in the frequently reported fear of having a heart attack on the street and being mistaken for a drunk and ignored.

Sexuality

The issue of sexuality comes up very often with these male veterans. It seems that most group members are well acquainted with the stories of John Garfield and Nelson Rockefeller, both of whom died while making love to a younger woman. "What a way to die" is the constant comment. However, after a bit of bravado a depressed mood prevails. What usually follows are discussion as to how medication affects the libido and complaints that doctors do not tell them what they can do. While attending a lecture on cardiovascular disease at a New York hospital I heard a physician discuss how, prior to discharge, he walks cardiac patients up a flight of stairs. He then turns to them and says, "By the way, walking up a flight of stairs is equivalent to sexual intercourse." At this lecture it was also pointed out that it is much more taxing and stressful for a person to have sex with an acquaintance as opposed to having it with a spouse or long-time girlfriend, which is more familiar and relaxing. Related to this, one patient in group pointed out how he and his wife have unhurried sex with a lot of consideration by the wife. This patient amusingly stated that he does not chase after buses either!

THE INFLUENCE OF A WOMAN IN THE GROUP

Since in our culture heart disease is associated with being male, problems arise when because of the disease a man "no longer functions physically as in the past" (Stein, 1983). Stein states that men benefit more from a mixed setting, in that they are able to personalize more and to express more of their feelings. In all-male group settings, Stein found, there was more concern with status and competition between members.

From my experience with the group described here, I found that when a woman veteran was present in a session, changes took place. For one, she would try to involve quiet members in the group (this almost never happened when only men were present). It also seemed that the men were more polite and tried to set a more positive tone for the group. However, in contrast to Stein, I did not find the men in my group to be particularly concerned with competition or status. This may be explained by the fact that the groups cited by Stein were mainly discussion and consciousness-raising groups, in which there is less intense preoccupation with issues around death and dying and the suffering of losses.

THE GROUP AS A SUPPORT SYSTEM

Many of the cardiac patients admitted to the hospital are here for cardiac catheterization and possible open heart surgery or bypass operations. The group members are very helpful to new members who are anxious about the upcoming surgery. Members who have undergone these procedures will describe them and usually minimize the risk factors, presenting the surgery as having given them a new lease on life. Even when members talk about two or more bypass operations that still occasion them a lot of pain, the general consensus is that surgery is essential for their survival.

When a patient in group complained that his wife has not been much help to him since his disability, since she never learned to drive the car and take care of financial matters, other members responded that they made sure that their spouses could handle these matters. These members then encouraged the patient by saying that it was not too late to teach his wife to handle more responsibilities and ease his stress. Support systems started in sessions seem to continue on the wards. Also noted is that patients become more intimate with each other and tend to spend more time together once they have been members of a group.

When asked about the group, male veterans feel for the most part that the sessions help them blow off steam and that they find them helpful. However, it appears that given their backgrounds they find it difficult to accept the group as psychotherapy per se; often they describe it as a B.S. session, though rewarding. For these men, mostly of working-class origin, this is a more familiar experience and thus more acceptable to them.

Interestingly, though possibly predictably, no matter how helpful and positive the previous session has been for the individual and the group, feelings are almost always expressed that the patient is "not up to it" the following week. This is due probably to frustration and feelings of powerlessness over being stuck in an acute care hospital with a life-threatening illness. It seems reasonable that the continuous dredging up, through group discussion, of these feelings is defended against by the healthy part of the patient. Seeing this as resistance is not the interpretation I would place on it. Since group members are, as I have mentioned, something of a captive audience (I do make rounds encouraging them to attend), I respect their refusal to attend without any confrontation on my part.

FUNCTIONS OF THE GROUP LEADER

In leading this group, I see the strengthening of coping skills and the reduction of anxieties as primary goals. Owing to the many losses suffered by these patients, these are not easy tasks to accomplish. The best one can hope for is to leave them feeling a little better about themselves, perhaps with the courage to go on with their lives as well as possible. Strengthening and improving support systems such as family and friends is another way of enriching their remaining years.

Coping skills can be strengthened by focusing on the positive —things that the group members are actually capable of. This will make them feel better about themselves and alleviate anxieties and feelings of helplessness and hopelessness. Reinforcing problem-solving skills is yet another approach that has proven helpful to these terminally ill, elderly veterans.

I sometimes raise the question of how they feel about the fact that I am the only one in the group who has never had a cardiac condition. A good time for this is after a member says something like, "Some people may have had a heart attack and don't know it," or "How do you feel working with us? Are you afraid?" Members at times feel protective of me, as when someone points out that I am a male and as vulnerable to heart attacks as they. I deal with the issues underlying such statements as empathically as possible. I express appreciation for the protectiveness implied and acknowledge the need to see me as powerful and less vulnerable than they. I consciously stay the idealized figure (Kohut, 1984) and neither confront nor dispute these feelings. To dwell on them, I feel, is not helpful for this population. Strengths rather than weaknesses should be stressed.

BURNOUTS IN GROUP LEADER AND PATIENTS

There are many reasons for the burnout syndrome, both in group leaders and patients. As previously suggested, the short-term open-ended group has very low status in the field of group psychotherapy owing to the instability of its ever changing membership, a feature which makes process and group development difficult (Schopler and Galinsky, 1984). This may leave the therapist with the feeling that this is not a "real" group experience, a feeling often magnified by the directive and concretized approach taken with such groups. Another factor that makes it difficult for the group leader to resist burnout is that this particular population, consisting mostly of very sick elderly males, puts the leader in touch with his own mortality. For example, while presenting this group to an ongoing in-service training group, I expressed at one point my feeling that "this could not happen to me." Fortunately, many of the sessions in this in-service training program were used, by myself and others, to get in touch with the difficulty of working with an acute care hospital population and the effect it has on us.

CONCLUSION

Short-term open-ended groups can be very helpful to the terminally ill population. The realization by group members that they are not alone in facing their physical limitations, and the empathy available from both the group leader and other members can both strengthen and comfort these highly vulnerable individuals. Above all, the group leader must strive to create a supportive environment for each individual in the group, regardless of that individual's particular coping style and defenses. While the reduction of anxiety generated by issues of death and loss should always be a goal, a member's need to cope by remaining consciously unaware of anxiety-producing material should always be respected. Indeed, this should be viewed not negatively, as resistance, but rather as helpful and necessary for the individual: he should not be expected to come to terms with his life-threatening illness other than through the style he has used, adaptively, all of his life.

REFERENCES

Burnside, I. M. (1978), *Working with the Elderly: Group Processes and Techniques.* North Scituate, Mass.: Duxbury Press.

Herr, J. J., & Weakland, J. H. (1979), *Counseling Elders and Their Families: Practical Techniques for Applied Gerontology.* New York: Springer.

Kohut, H. (1984), *How Does Analysis Cure?* Chicago: University of Chicago Press.

Lipton, H., & Walter, S. (1971), The social worker as mediator on a hospital ward. In: *The Practice of Group Work,* ed. W. Schwartz & S. R. Zalba. New York: Columbia University Press, pp. 97–121.

Schopler, J. H., & Galinsky, M. J. (1984), Meeting practice needs: Conceptualizing the open-ended group. *Social Work with Groups,* 7:3–21.

Slavson, S. R. (1964), *A Textbook in Analytic Group Psychotherapy.* New York: International Universities Press.

Spiegel, D., & Yalom, I. D. (1978), A support group for dying patients. *Internat. J. Group Psychother.,* 28:233–246.

Stein, T. S. (1983), An overview of men's group. *Social Work with Groups*, 6:17–26.
Weiner, M. B., Brok, A. J., & Snadowsky, A. M. (1978), *Working with the Aged*. Englewood Cliffs, N.J.: Prentice-Hall.
Weisman, A. D. (1972), *On Dying and Denying: A Psychiatric Study of Terminality*. New York: Behavioral Publications.
Yalom, I. D. (1975), *The Theory and Practice of Group Psychotherapy*. New York: Basic Books.

13

Group Psychotherapy with the Elderly in the State Hospital

DAVID BIENENFELD, M.D.

Despite the impact of nearly three decades of deinstitutionalization of the mentally ill, a large number of elderly individuals continue to reside in state mental hospitals or similar facilities. Major changes in resources and philosophy have mandated a concomitant shift in emphasis from custodial to rehabilitative services. The use of group treatment for the institutionalized elderly is not a new concept, but most of the focus until recently has been on such task-centered groups as orientation groups and music groups (Busse and Blazer, 1980; Verwoerdt, 1981; Kalson, 1982).

Psychotherapists in general are beginning to overcome traditional prejudices about the usefulness of psychotherapy in the elderly (e.g., Wolff, 1963); group therapists are currently exploring the particular character of group psychotherapy with this population (Berland and Poggi, 1979). In state hospitals, where the role of psychotherapy is not firmly established at all, group psychotherapy represents a new frontier (Meltzer, 1982).

This chapter draws on the findings of others as well as my own experience in leading a psychotherapy group in a state hospital, the Pauline Warfield Lewis Center in Cincinnati, Ohio. This group has been meeting regularly for over five years, coled by the author for most of that time. The cotherapist is a female occupational therapist. Group members are black and white men and women drawn from each of the four wards of the geriatric section of the hospital. They range in age from late fifties to late seventies, and carry many diagnoses, including major depression, bipolar disorder, schizophrenia, and various personality disorders. Group size has varied from four to nine members. Patients are referred to the group by the treatment team of the home ward, and are screened by one of the cotherapists. Criteria for admission are: (1) the patient must have some history in the past two years of a degree of interpersonal involvement or social adaptation; (2) the patient must be willing to attend the group for at least four sessions as a trial (no one is ordered to attend); and (3) the patient must have no cognitive impairment that would prohibit his comprehension and participation in the group. The group meets weekly for sixty minutes.

STRUCTURE

These structural characteristics represent choices that will vary among groups, depending on such factors as resources, environment, and objectives. The use of cotherapists can be technically complicated (Rutan and Stone, 1984), and may be incompatible with the style and personality of even a skilled group therapist. Busse and Blazer (1980), however, point out some advantages of the cotherapy model. Each therapist can clarify and refine the interventions of the other, a function of immense value in a setting where the patients' capacities for abstraction are usually limited. A male-female pair of leaders promotes the emergence of manifestations of parental transference, a useful regression which often requires facilitation in the elderly (Bienenfeld, 1985). As discussed below, the group in an institution is highly valued by its members as a source of information. Coleaders of different professional backgrounds can thus bring to the group a wide array of knowledge.

There is considerable difference of opinion regarding the age distribution of group members. Some, most notably Butler (1975), advocate groups including young as well as old members, holding that younger adults can learn from the experience of the elderly, who can then feel a sense of accomplishment and value. Further, this heterogeneity accentuates the longitudinal impact of the life cycle for all parties. Others, including Verwoerdt (1981) and Busse and Blazer (1980), maintain that geriatric groups should be segregated because their styles and issues are quite age-specific. In the state hospital, several additional factors tend to favor age homogeneity. Geriatric sections are often administratively and even physically separate from other sections, and have social communities that are quite different.

In many states, governmental pressures have shaped the adult sections of these institutions to include mostly severely ill patients who are discharged quickly, while geriatric patients may be less floridly ill and stay longer. Thus, age-integrated groups could have difficulty finding common goals. Older patients may also experience their younger counterparts as threatening, to an extent that may undermine cohesion beyond the capacity of any therapist to repair.

Heterogeneity by diagnosis is almost universally accepted (Busse and Blazer, 1980; Bloor, 1981; Katz, 1983). The group can thereby become representative of its members' social community. More variable are the criteria for group membership. The state hospital rarely offers the therapist the opportunity to hold to restrictive criteria for inclusion (Kalson, 1982). However, recent advances in group theory and technique enable him to compose a group based mainly on exclusion (Meltzer, 1982). At a minimum, one must exclude those who have an organic incapacity to understand or participate, those who are unmanageably disruptive, and those who are unworkably lacking in motivation. Beyond these minimal criteria, the therapist can consider selection based on personality traits, communicative styles, imminence of discharge, etc., depending on the available population, the therapist's preferences, and the goals of the group.

GOALS

Central to these decisions, and to the conduct of the group therapy, is the establishment of goals for the group (Yalom, 1983; Rutan and Stone, 1984). The age of the members and the institutional setting certainly place some restrictions on the range of feasible goals. For example, fully independent functioning in the community is rarely a credible option for these group members, and goals relating to such an outcome would be inappropriate. Nonetheless, there is a large array of goals from which the therapist may choose, including constructive life review (Butler, 1975), improvement of interpersonal relationships and social integration, amelioration of symptoms of depression and paranoia (Kalson, 1982), or arrival at effective problem-solving strategies (Verwoerdt, 1981). Goals devised in the service of the facility may include promoting discharge and diminishing management difficulties (Berland and Poggi, 1979; Kalson, 1982). Yalom (1983) points out that whatever goals the therapist may entertain a priori, the working goals must be negotiated and clarified within the group itself, so that each member has a sense of ownership in goals valuable to himself.

THEMES

Many of the themes that emerge are common to all forms of psychotherapy with the elderly, such as loss, nostalgia, and fear of illness and death (Berland and Poggi, 1979; Busse and Blazer, 1980; Verwoerdt, 1981). Issues of hostility and competition, power and authority, and fear of change are common to all groups, and are no less evident in this setting. The institutional environment, however, alters not only the manifestations but the very nature of these issues (Yalom, 1983).

In one session, for example, our group began discussing evening activities on the wards.

Doris: Why do they make us go to bed at eight o'clock? Isn't that awfully early?

Carol: Eight? We don't have to be in bed until nine on our ward.

D.B.: Who makes you go to bed at eight?

Doris: Well, that's the curfew, isn't it?

Gus: You don't have to, but everybody does. You get your medicine and go to bed. There's nothing to do.

J.M. (cotherapist): Actually, the hospital rules say you can be up until at least eleven.

Doris: Eleven? Oh, my! I didn't know that.

J.M.: Do you think you would be able to ask to stay up later if you wanted to?

Doris: Oh, no! They would think I was being sassy. They'd just say, "Go back to your room."

(When the therapists attempted to explore Doris's transferential assumptions, Doris changed subjects, with widespread cooperation from the other members. Later in the same session, however, the issue was elaborated.)

Martha: Ms. Brown tells us we have to be back on the ward at seven, but I know the rules say we're allowed to be outside until eight in the summer. It just makes it more convenient for her.

D.B.: It seems the rules are being bent for the benefit of the staff, at some cost to you?

Martha: Yes, but I'd never mention it to her.

D.B.: Why not?

Martha: I wouldn't want to cross her. She's done so many favors for all of us, this doesn't seem like a lot for her to ask.

This discussion begins with references to authority that could be part of almost any psychotherapy group. In this context, however, the therapists are obliged to investigate first whether the restrictions are primarily internal (Doris's) or external (the system's). The group can concede that the restrictions are not primarily an effect of non-negotiable hospital rules. However, they cannot accept the therapists' naive notion that each patient can simply assert himself without consequence. Doris imagines that such an attempt will be met with resistance or retaliation (not altogether imaginary), while Martha points out that, even without retaliation, group members live in a system where one goes along to get along.

Problems of personal autonomy and responsibility thus take on new meaning in an environment that sets very real limits on both. Privacy of property, person, and information is a matter of tremendous concern to these patients, in a way that transcends the familiar worry about sharing with a group. Patients constantly work over the question of what a "caregiver" is and should be—whose well-being is served, whose wishes addressed.

BOUNDARIES

Since the environment so forcefully shapes the issues with which the group members struggle, it follows naturally that management and violations of group boundaries assume tremendous importance in understanding the group process. On a concrete level, these patients have limited control over their own schedules. While absences from an outpatient group for medical clinic appointments or haircuts are generally viewed in the context of resistances, here such absences may instead serve to highlight the members' real or perceived lack of control over their own activities. Open discussion of such absences allows the members to examine what choices they have, what rights they can exercise. Those who are "left behind" by the absent member can use these boundary violations as an opportunity to reflect on their own feelings of disappointment, jealousy, relief, or resentment. Similarly, physical illnesses are common. By focusing on the effect of the sick member's absence from the group, the therapist can help patients deal in a near displacement, with sensations of fear or threat that might be too potent to examine directly.

In most other contexts, contact between members outside the group may appropriately be viewed as a stretching or breaking of boundary rules. These patients, however, live together (Yalom, 1983). In the group discussed here, such contact is overtly identified as a goal of treatment. Members describe their interactions and are encouraged to examine factors that facilitate or inhibit social engagement. Feedback is obtained from the other party, allowing members to become aware of unwarranted and counterproductive assumptions they carry into relationships. These observations are then generalized to other encounters.

By the same token, group therapists in state hospitals usually have other jobs that bring them into contact with group members (Yalom, 1983). These outside contacts can range from field trips to civil commitment hearings and are often quite different in character from the group psychotherapy sessions. The discrepancies, to which patients can be remarkably sensitive, are acknowledged and subsequently used to help patients differentiate individuals from the jobs they hold.

One particular manifestation of this duality of roles is a concern over confidentiality (Yalom, 1983). Doris was a patient on the author's ward. After discussing in group an upcoming visit with her daughter, Doris approached me privately on the ward and recounted some delusional ideas about the daughter, asking that I tell no one. I explained I would need to share her concerns with the treatment team, but failed to make any mention of the psychotherapy group. At the next group meeting, Doris related in detail her belief that the priest told his secretary what Doris told him in confession. The therapists took the opportunity to elicit members' notions about confidentiality in the group, ranging from a belief in our absolute secrecy to a cynical conviction that everything quickly became public knowledge. Even after we clarified the conditional confidentiality of group material, they kept the fantasies in mind in other discussions of trust and reliability.

Bloor (1981) discusses eloquently some of the paradoxes arising from group treatment in a therapeutic community. These paradoxes consistently confront the institutional group therapist. Some have already been touched on. For example, group members are encouraged to explore areas of autonomy and personal choice. Yet staff in most state hospitals will tend to respond more favorably to "cooperation," which is often inconsistent with autonomy.

Perhaps the central paradox confronting patients is that the reward for adaptive functioning in the milieu is discharge from it, a far more daunting prospect than termination from an outpatient group or even discharge from an acute care hospital. The patient culture labels it as "crazy" not to want to leave the hospital. It is here that the psychotherapy group can be invaluable as a forum for identifying ambivalence about the hospital community.

At the last group meeting before her discharge, Carol told the other members: "I've been here off and on for forty-five years. I've never thought of this place as home because I always wanted to remember my real home on the outside. But this hospital has been *like* home. I've learned a lot and made some wonderful friends, including some of you. I'm glad to go, but I'll miss you and I thank you for your help."

TECHNIQUE

Those who practice group psychotherapy with the elderly are aware that they must constantly reevaluate all assumptions about technique. The most common admonition is that the therapist be "active" (e.g., Foster and Foster, 1983). The meaning of activity, however, is rarely defined. Elderly participants in psychotherapy, even in chronic care institutions, need not be considered incapable of introspection and self-examination. The therapist who hurries to give advice or to offer soothing comments to the troubled member may be forfeiting an opportunity to foster change and growth. Being active more productively involves being aware of issues likely to be at work in the group at a particular time, so as to be sensitive to near displacements of these issues and assist the group in examining them. Thus one is simultaneously evaluating age-independent functions of group process (e.g., the effects of an absence or the entry of a new member) and life-cycle manifestations (e.g., coming to grips with one's own mortality). Anticipation without prejudice allows the therapist to keep the group's attention focused. Within that focus, patients can often tolerate a considerable amount of frustration and conflict without requiring the therapist's interference.

Yalom (1983) has argued eloquently for the applicability of a "here-and-now" approach to inpatient group psychotherapy. The relevance of the rationale is unaffected by the age of the members or the nature of the hospital. In brief, the pathology that is likely to be central to the therapeutic goals is for the most part interpersonally based. Further, that pathology is reenacted in the group setting. Past history can be used to make sense of the presence of patterns of perception and response, but finding more adaptive patterns must be practiced in the present. The therapist points out the patterns to the group and facilitates understanding of the reasons the patterns exist in the first place, their maladaptive consequences in the present, and alternative patterns of relating.

Rather than point out only the pathological patterns of perception and interaction, the therapist is well advised to promote and encourage patterns that are adaptive (Liberman, 1970). Institutional patients are accustomed to receiving orders (however polite) and criticism, but are often starved for positive feedback when they have acted or spoken in a desirable fashion. When group members communicate directly with each other, rather than giving speeches or addressing the therapists exclusively, this action and its positive consequences should be noted publicly. Acknowledgment of ambivalent feelings and overt evidence of caring for other members can be dealt with similarly.

When Martha complained that the departure of one patient on her ward left her without company, the therapist asked if she might spend time with someone from another ward, to which Martha shrugged. When he further asked about members of this group, she replied that no one went anywhere. Pearl countered, "I'll go out with you," but received only a polite nod. Subsequently, members asked if anyone had heard from Carol, who had been discharged a few weeks earlier. No one had, and the therapist noted that Carol, at her last group session, had asked the members to come and visit. With some encouragement, the members clarified that what they wanted was a more specific invitation. Pearl wanted to be sure that she was truly wanted and valued, not merely being treated politely.

Soon afterward Martha remarked on how an aide on her ward failed to notice how active and useful she was. Before the therapist could make the connection, Pearl said, "Martha, do you want to go to the shopping center with me this Wednesday?" Martha agreed, this time with animation. The therapist underlined for the group how Pearl had used the message of her own feelings about Carol, and how helpful her action was for Martha.

Loss is one of the most frequently noted themes in geriatric groups. Early in my experience, I sought to help my groups "work through" these losses with appropriate grieving and recovery. Two factors interfered, however. First, the patients would distance themselves from attempted reflections about their feelings of pain, saying, "It doesn't bother me; I'm used to it." Second, the deaths, the illnesses, the departures of staff members, and other losses were occurring so frequently that it seemed impossible to recover from one before another was upon them. It turned out to be most productive to attend to the members' messages about the ubiquity and chronicity of losses. Acknowledgment of their existential vulnerability allowed the patients to examine their ambivalence about lost objects, and their inner fears. It also allowed them to identify the strengths of their most resilient and adaptive responses.

Since the group members are institutional patients, it would be misleading to imply that all discussions are at a coherent, sophisticated level. More often than not, work begins at a concrete level—daily events, food, etc. By tracking the emotional content and making educated guesses about symbolism, the therapist attempts to discover the meaning of the story. While attempts may be made to translate these messages, such activity is not always necessary. Katz's notions about the noninterpretation of metaphors in some groups (1983) are often relevant here. If the therapist can follow the meaning, the group can often discuss the message at arm's length. They can discuss "what-if" wrinkles, and draw generalizable conclusions from the fable they have created.

In the state hospital (perhaps even more than in other systems of comparable size) obtaining accurate information is a difficult task. Rumor, secrecy, and contradiction are commonplace. Patients come to trust the group therapists and look to them for accurate answers to questions about the system. Direct answers should be provided when possible, but the opportunity should be used to explore the members' use of other resources (including one another). Equally productive are the group's responses to situations in which the therapists are themselves confused by the system.

Often, of course, state hospital patients will become psychotic. The therapist's dual role here is to limit the destructive impact and to help the group understand the disruptive behavior (Meltzer, 1982). In the course of group development, the leader becomes aware of how much psychotic communication the group can tolerate before it becomes destructive. It should be part of the group contract that patients may be asked to take a break from the group when their emotional states prevent their effective participation. In each such case, clear criteria should be given—to both the individual and the group—for return to the group. Groups can learn a great deal from observing the therapist's handling of psychotic communication, and from their own responses as observers or objects of the behavior. The member who has become disruptive can make a valuable contribution by discussing the experience after recompensating.

SUMMARY

The state hospital setting offers opportunities to help elderly patients with group therapy at an ambitious level. Goals must be established first that are consistent with the capacities and resources of the patients. Themes that arise in therapy are not dissimilar from those heard in any psychotherapy group, but are shaped in their manifestations not only by the age of the group members, but also by the influences of the hospital setting. Autonomy and expression which are promoted in the group may be discouraged in the larger environment. Confidentiality is more than a passing worry. The nature of the patients in such a group mandates flexibility in technique. The therapist must actively anticipate issues and be ready to intervene so as to promote group work. Adjustments must be made to accommodate the occasional emergence of psychosis in group members.

REFERENCES

Berland, D. I., & Poggi, R. (1979), Expressive group psychotherapy with the aging. *Internat. J. Group Psychother.*, 29:87–108.
Bienenfeld, D. (1985), The two-way street: Aspects of regression in psychotherapy with aging patients. *Amer. J. Psychother.*, 39:86–93.
Bloor, M. J. (1981), Therapeutic paradox: The patient culture and the formal treatment programme in a therapeutic community. *Brit. J. Med. Psychol.*, 54:359–369.
Busse, E. W., & Blazer, D. G. (1980), *Handbook of Geriatric Psychiatry*. New York: Van Nostrand Reinhold.
Butler, R. N. (1975), Psychiatry and the elderly: An overview. *Amer. J. Psychiat.*, 132:893–900.
Foster, J. R., & Foster, R. R. (1983), Group psychotherapy with the old and aged. In: *Comprehensive Group Psychotherapy*, ed. H. I. Kaplan & B. J. Sadock. Baltimore: Williams & Wilkins, pp. 269–277.
Kalson, L. (1982), Group therapy with the aged. In: *Group Psychotherapy and Counselling with Special Populations*, ed. M. Seligman. Baltimore: University Park Press, pp. 77–98.

Katz, G. A. (1983), The noninterpretation of metaphors in psychiatric hospital groups. *Internat. J. Group Psychother.*, 33:53–67.

Liberman, R. (1970), A behavioral approach to group dynamics: I. Reinforcement and prompting of cohesiveness in group therapy. *Behavior Therapy*, 1:141–175.

Meltzer, S. W. (1982), Group analytic approaches to psychotic patients in an institutional setting. *Amer. J. Psychoanal.*, 42:357–362.

Rutan, J. S., & Stone, W. N. (1984), *Psychodynamic Group Psychotherapy*. Toronto: Collamore Press.

Verwoerdt, A. (1981), *Clinical Geropsychiatry*. Baltimore: Williams & Wilkins.

Wolff, K. (1963), *Geriatric Psychiatry*. Springfield, Ill.: Thomas.

Yalom, I. D. (1983), *Inpatient Group Psychotherapy*. New York: Basic Books.

14

Selecting Family Caregivers of Alzheimer Patients for Group Psychotherapy

MIRIAM K. ARONSON, Ed.D.

Dementing illness, the most common cause of mental impairment among older persons, currently affects four million Americans and is a major public health problem. Alzheimer's disease is the most common form of dementing illness, accounting for the majority of cases. One-third of dementia victims are so impaired that they can no longer manage without assistance in the simplest routine activities of daily living. If one estimates that each dementia victim may have three close family members, the number of persons affected escalates rapidly. Alzheimer's disease and other dementias pose a threat to the afflicted person, to his family and friends, and ultimately to our society (Aronson, 1984).

Alzheimer's disease is the fourth leading cause of death in adults, accounting for at least 120,000 deaths annually (Katzman, 1976). While this statistic is significant, it does not begin to suggest the breadth of human suffering involved. There is probably no greater affliction than for a person to deteriorate inch by inch over a period of years—perhaps seven to ten or more—as family and friends stand helplessly by. Spouses have described the experience as living in a state of limbo—neither wives nor widows, neither husbands nor widowers. Others talk of suddenly living with strangers.

Family members provide 80 percent of the day-to-day care at home. For every demented person in a nursing home (and some 60 percent of nursing home residents are demented) there are several of similar incapacity residing at home. Not the actual degree of intellectual, social, or physical impairment but social and financial factors—who is available to care for the patient, how much time and energy the family caregiver can expend, how much money is available for purchasing outside services when these are needed—are likely to determine whether and when a dementia patient is placed in a long-term care facility.

Alzheimer's disease has a long and protracted course—five to seven years according to DSM–III, but often much longer in our clinical experience. During this time there are substantial emotional burdens imposed on family caregivers, in addition to the need to provide twenty-four-hour care and supervision (Zarit, Reever, and Bach-Peterson, 1980). There are several unique features of Alzheimer's disease which heighten this emotional burden. First, the patient's physical intactness presents a dilemma in the face of cognitive decline. It is a constant struggle for family members to deal rationally with the ever widening discrepancy between appearance and function. Second, denial is perpetuated by the insidious and unrelenting progression of a condition that has no identifiable "bouts of illness." How can someone be "sick" when he always looks so well? Third, the presence of variable insight can be devastating for the caregiver. A usually mute patient who spontaneously says something appropriate can confuse the caregiver. Fourth, lack of communication and feedback for the caregiver makes providing constant care a thankless task.

Services available for the dementia patient are limited primarily by the fact that little or no third-party reimbursement is available for ongoing care through Medicare or private health insurance. While Medicaid, the needs-based government-paid system for the medically indigent, may pay for some needed services, most persons do not meet this program's financial eligibility criteria. Hence, despite the government's large expenditures for nursing home care, these funds are provided for only a small fraction of dementia patients. *Most dementia patients are cared for at home by family caregivers.* At this time, the reimbursement system provides little or no incentive or relief for these caregivers.

The intense and sustained emotional burdens of caregivers exact their toll. Caregiver burden is a construct that has been sparsely researched. It has been reported that decreased social supports are correlated with feelings of increased burden (Zarit, Reever, and Bach-Peterson, 1980). Stress-related illnesses are more prevalent among caregivers than would be expected, although this phenomenon is not well studied. Further, depression in this group has been found to be pervasive (Eisdorfer, Kennedy, Wisnieski, and Cohen, 1983; Steuer, 1984).

Denial is one of the central issues in working with family caregivers; ultimately it must be confronted so that necessary planning and decision-making can be accomplished. Families tend to deny and cover up for their loved one's deficits. While denial may be helpful in the early phases of dealing with this catastrophic illness, it falters as the disease progresses and deficits must be confronted. How much can a caregiver deny when she says, "Put your socks on," and the patient puts them on his hands? It should be noted that patients deny or don't recognize their problem and are therefore poor historians for treating professionals (Reifler, Larson, and Hanley, 1982).

Anger is fostered and re-created by the frustrations the caregiver encounters in being with the patient—perseveration, comprehension difficulties, inappropriate or embarrassing behaviors. Further, the lack of services, the expense involved in obtaining them, or a sense of hopelessness no matter what services are obtained are factors in promoting and perpetuating caregiver anger. This anger heightens the potential for conflict and for abuse as well. Providing a means of expressing this anger and thus decreasing the potential for conflict is thus an important therapeutic strategy.

With the escalating incapacity of the Alzheimer patient, performance of accustomed activities and roles becomes increasingly difficult. Early in the course of the disease the patient may experience difficulty in traveling around without getting lost or perhaps difficulty in managing finances (paying bills or balancing a checkbook). As these difficulties develop it becomes necessary for the "well" spouse or other caregiver to assume these responsibilities. The wife who never drove may now have to learn how—one of our program participants got her driver's license at age sixty-nine. A daughter or son may have to become a parent to a father or mother. These role reversals challenge the abilities of the individuals involved and change the homeostasis of long-standing relationships. The denial we observe is probably perpetuated by the fear of these very changes—the dependent woman, who now has a dependent husband, is faced with the need for her to exercise control in a deteriorating situation.

Dementing illness involves prolonged irresolvable grief. The cognitive, functional, and eventual physical decline of the patient is inexorable. Ultimately the person residing in the body of the victim becomes entirely different, but still the living body stays on, often for a very long time. Actual death may occur years after the victim's decline into nonfunctional existence, and thus inherently there is a prolonged mourning process.

Because of the similarity of dementia symptoms to mental illness, and because dementia and behavioral and affective symptoms often coexist (Reifler, Larson, and Hanley, 1982), help-seeking is often delayed. In a recent study (Aronson, Gaston, and Merriam, 1984) the average time elapsed between the onset of cognitive symptoms and the seeking of a diagnostic workup was more than four years in a cohort of ninety-nine dementia patients. At the time of diagnosis, no matter how advanced the course of the disease, and no matter how stressed the caregiver at that point, caregivers generally do not perceive themselves as patients. They often deny that their loved one will ever get "that bad." They say, "I can handle it—if it doesn't get any worse," and do not seek help until a time of crisis. Typically, the first call for help is one requesting concrete services such as a psychiatrist for the patient, a geriatrician for medical care, a neurologist for another opinion, or a drug research program. Often even this information gets filed away without any action, as the spouse may remain immobilized by denial for a long time.

It is usually a crisis situation that finally brings the caregiver to seek help. The crisis that usually occurs earliest in the course of the disease revolves around finances. A mother may suddenly have received an eviction notice for nonpayment of rent, though her daughter discovers she has thousands of dollars' worth of uncashed checks in her pocketbook. A husband has always taken good care of the finances, but suddenly checks are bouncing because he's paid the same bill several times, made a deposit to the wrong account, or forgotten to make a deposit at all. Not only must the caregiver now admit that there's a problem, but must act quickly to remedy it. The dreaded role reversals often start here, and are often not easy. A mother may become paranoid and accuse her daughter of having stolen her checks. A husband may accuse his wife of taking away his money or of "butting into his affairs." In an extreme case a husband may call the police regarding "theft" or may even file for divorce (as happened in one case). The significant other is devastated and often seeks assistance at this point. Even then, the caregiver may get the support needed to work through the immediate crisis but then reject further help.

A second crisis often involves termination of the patient's driving an automobile. Another crisis may occur when the spouse can no longer manage the patient without outside assistance. The willingness to admit needing help is pivotal, but what often causes the caregiver to finally realize that the situation is getting out of control is embarrassment. When husbands or wives wander out of the house naked, caregivers are faced with retrieving them. When the patient is at the store and takes an item without paying for it, it is the caregiver who must explain. These embarrassing experiences may drive spouses to seek supportive help for themselves. If not, some caregivers' achievement of "patient" status for themselves becomes painfully evident: states of being overwhelmed; prolonged sleeplessness leading to physical exhaustion; social isolation due to withdrawal of family and friends; clinically significant depression; and physical illness.

Once they recognize their own need for help, caregivers may seek help in many ways: they may ask the family doctor for medication; they may attend self-help groups; they may seek individual therapy; they may seek group therapy; or they may seek day care or other respite or even nursing home placement for the patient.

Although families are generally woefully underserved at this time, one of the more widely available resources for families is group programs—support groups or other group modalities. At this time, the group modalities available are highly variable in terms of model, auspices, and quality of service. Essentially, there are educational, therapeutic, supportive, and self-help models (Aronson and Yatzkan, 1984). The educational model is often either a time-limited small group program with a heavy didactic component and limited opportunity for discussion; or a larger "audience" topical session with a formal presentation with or without opportunity for interchange in the group as a whole or in smaller discussion groups. The therapeutic model is a professionally led group whose members have a common problem, i.e., the dementia of their relative. Similar groups may be a little broader in focus, serving caregivers of the "frail elderly." Support groups may be agency- or community-based, may have a combined professional and lay leadership, and may be organized around certain commonalities, such as caring at home, placement in a long-term care facility, or bereavement. They may be open or closed, time-limited or open-ended. Self-help groups for families of dementia victims are most often under the auspices of chapters of the national Alzheimer's Disease and Related Disorders Association, a voluntary health organization established in 1979. These may be "leaderless," may be led by a lay family member or volunteer professional, or may have a combination of family and professional leadership.

Group sponsorship may vary from community to community, but the educational and self-help support models are probably most often under the auspices of chapters or affiliates of the Alzheimer's Disease and Related Disorders Association, although hospitals, family agencies, nursing homes, mental health centers, church groups, or aging groups may also provide sponsorship. Therapeutic groups may be services of family agencies or groups, mental health agencies, hospital clinics, or private practitioners.

As definitions of groups, models, meeting formats, group composition, and leadership vary, so too do the quantity and quality of the services provided. For the most part groups may be a vital link with a supportive network for the caregiver; however, the variations mentioned may be responsible for widespread disparities in focus and quality (Schmall, 1984).

Given these facts, the question arises, who make the best group participants? Obviously, this would be applicable only to groups where there is an opportunity to select members—not the case in most self-help support groups—and is possible or practical only where there is professional leadership.

As in any group program, potential participants should have at least one screening interview. At this time the therapist will have an opportunity to assess affect, level of interest, personal characteristics, interpersonal skills, and type of service needed. Additionally, the interview provides an opportunity to introduce the program and to discuss and clarify expectations. Following is a discussion of some aspects of the caregiver or patient which merit consideration in selecting caregivers for group.

Diagnosis. The patient's having had a careful and reasonably accurate diagnosis is important. It matters not whether the diagnosis is Alzheimer's disease or multi-infarct dementia or a mixed dementia. The important factor is that there is a progressive and irreversible dementing process. The caregiver group cannot and should not be a place for speculation or armchair diagnosis.

Setting of the patient. Those who care for patients at home have different needs in terms of management information and assistance with making decisions regarding obtaining help, respite, and perhaps placement. Those whose loved ones now reside in a nursing home may have common concerns about nursing home policies or practices and about the loneliness and perhaps guilt that they are feeling.

Socioeconomic status and gender. These do not seem to be important variables in group composition; rather, it is the level of functional impairment of the patient that seems the most important determinant. Relatives of newly diagnosed patients may have little in common with relatives of patients in nursing homes.

Relationship to the patient. Children's concerns are different from the concerns of spouses. Likewise, caregiving family members may have needs different from those of noncaregiving relatives.

Age. A forty-five-year-old spouse with teenage children may have needs very different from those of a spouse of seventy-five. Age per se, however, is a poor determinant, as persons of similar age may have very dissimilar needs and interests.

Openness. As in any group, members need to share and must be willing to work. Commitment to the group program is also most important. Those who are merely "shopping" for services, i.e., running from institution to institution, probably will not sustain their participation in the program. Those who are secretive about their loved one's problem will also be less likely to benefit from participation.

Serious psychopathology. This should be screened out. Some persons tend to use the Alzheimer's disease of their relative as an excuse for longstanding pathology. All groups are not suitable for all persons and vice versa. Some persons may require individual treatment. In addition, persons who become clinically depressed may require medication as well as psychotherapy.

Relationships. The illness of a spouse usually strains good relationships and exacerbates bad ones. In the selection process, careful attention should be paid to the existence of violence or other abuse. In cases where abuse is suspected, the group is probably the wrong setting for the caregiver, at least initially. It should be noted that in relationships where the couple was merged, there will be resistance or even an inability to change (Steuer, 1984).

Knowledge. Those who know that the state of the art is good long-term management, but not cure or even dramatic "fixes" of any kind, will be better group members than those seeking a "magic pill." While one of the goals of the group is overcoming denial, the presence of excessive and overwhelming denial will prevent good group participation.

From the above, it may be concluded that some amount of homogeneity is desirable. Clearly this is true; however it may be impractical or even impossible in some settings—rural areas, for example, where group participants must travel long distances and may be unable to attend on a frequent basis. Further, dementia patients who are cared for at home span a broad spectrum of functional and behavioral impairments. While discussion about very impaired patients may be upsetting for some, the opportunity to get comfort from "someone who has been there" may prove invaluable for others. Moreover, caregivers tend to use groups around crisis points in the illness and may thus be unwilling to make more than a very limited time commitment.

Alzheimer's disease is a great social leveler, reducing the quality of lives of patients and their caregivers to bare survival activities. Group modalities, probably the most common form of help for caregivers, must provide, regardless of format, a combination of information and education with support and therapy; they must be goal-oriented; and they must deal with crises as they emerge. The selection of caregiver participants should be based on the variables outlined above. Research into their value as firm predictors of successful participation, however, is yet to be done.

REFERENCES

Aronson, M. (1982), Alzheimer's disease: An overview. *J. Western Gerontolog. Soc.*, 7:6–7

——— (1984), Alzheimer's and other dementias: A major public health problem. *Carrier Foundation Letter*, 102.

——— Gaston, P., & Merriam, A. (1984), Depression associated with depression. *J. Western Gerontolog. Soc.*, 9(2):49–51.

——— Levin, G. and Lipkowitz, R. (1984), A community-based family/patient group program for Alzheimer's disease. *Gerontologist*, 24:(4):339–342.

——— Yatzkan, E. (1984), The emerging support group movement. *Aging*, 347:3–9.

Barnes, R. F., Raskind, M. A., Scott, M., and Murphy, C. (1981), Problems of families caring for Alzheimer patients: Use of a support group. *J. Amer. Geriatrics Soc.*, 29(2):80–85.

Eisdorfer, C., Kennedy, G., Wisnieski, W., & Cohen, D. (1983), Depression and attributional style in families coping with the stress of caring for a relative with Alzheimer's disease. *Gerontologist*, 23:115–116.

Katzman, R. (1976), The prevalence and malignancy of Alzheimer's disease, a major killer. *Arch. Neurol.*, 33:217–218.

Reifler, B. V., Larson, E., & Hanley, R. (1982), Coexistence of cognitive impairment and depression in geriatric outpatients. *Amer. J. Psychiat.*, 139:623–626.

Schmall, V. (1984), What makes a support group good. *J. Western Gerontolog. Soc.*, 9(2):64–67.

Steuer, J. (1984), Working with caregivers. *J. Western Gerontolog. Soc.*, 9(2):56–58.

Zarit, S. H., Reever, K. E., & Bach-Peterson, J. (1980), Relatives of the impaired elderly: Correlates of feelings of burden. *Gerontologist*, 20(6):649–654.

15

Group Therapy with Confused and Disoriented Elderly People

SIDNEY R. SAUL, Ed.D., C.S.W., A.C.S.W.

Within the past several years, the plight of elderly people suffering from confusion and disorientation (and the concurrent suffering of their families) has become highly visible. It has been estimated that over 50 percent of the institutionalized elderly in the United States (about one million people) and another 1.3 million elderly people residing in the community are so affected (Trubo, 1984).

Attention has been directed to six major causes of confusion and disorientation in people over sixty-five (National Institute on Aging, 1980). These factors may be organic or functional and may occur singly or in combination. Functional causes include (1) the use of drugs, both prescription and nonprescription, and drug interactions (HCOA, 1983); (2) depression, a common but often overlooked condition which may be related to the losses attendant on aging (Reisberg, 1982); and (3) malnutrition, another common and often overlooked condition, which may be related to financial circumstances as well as to social isolation. These three factors are suspected of causing as much as 60 percent of the disorientation and confusion among elderly people, much of which is considered reversible. The three major organic conditions most commonly identified are (4) Alzheimer's disease and related disorders; (5) stroke; and (6) multi-infarct dementia.

Much attention has been focused on Alzheimer's disease. This illness, termed the "silent epidemic," was first isolated by Dr. Alois Alzheimer in 1906. At that time his patients were relatively younger people, and the disease was designated as "a rare disease of middle-aged people." Not until the late 1970s did the medical profession

197

discover that Alzheimer's disease, though indeed rare among younger people, was all too common among the older population (Reisberg, 1981).

The illness is silent. Its beginnings often go unnoticed, as the person begins to forget small and unimportant things. But as the neurotransmitters of the brain develop plaque and nerve fibers become tangled, the course of Alzheimer's disease is relentless. It becomes progressively worse, causes increased cognitive loss, and eventually results in death after seven to ten years (Mace and Rabens, 1981).

THE GROUP PROGRAMS

This chapter describes two therapy groups for confused and disoriented elderly people, most of whom have been diagnosed as having Alzheimer's disease. One group comprises inpatients residing in a skilled nursing facility (Kingsbridge Heights Manor, Bronx, N.Y.). These patients tend to suffer from a combination of physical illnesses (in addition to Alzheimer's disease) which contribute to their confusion. Depression, an almost inevitable concomitant of institutional living, is also an important dimension of their diagnoses. The other group is composed of outpatients in a community mental health center (Community Mental Health Center–Maimonides Medical Center, Brooklyn, New York), and has the unique feature of involving their caregivers. The members of this group tend to be in better physical health than the nursing home residents, except for the diagnosis of Alzheimer's disease. All are ambulatory. Some, like the nursing home patients, are depressed, especially those in the earlier stages of the disease, as they tend to be more aware of their cognitive loss.

General Purposes of the Group Programs

For the patients. Both groups are meant to (1) offer peer experiences and emotional support through group interaction and supportive, compassionate group leadership; (2) stimulate, encourage, and support intellectual and social capacities, using the group to accept varied levels of individual offerings through the use of available memory, the motivation of cognitive functioning via discussion, question and answer, and problem solving, and the fostering of socialization through the group experience; (3) affirm and confirm a sense of individual identity, which tends to become diffused for a person in a confused and disoriented state; (4) offer an ego-supportive experience; (5) counter the depression that accompanies confusion and disorientation; and (6) enhance the quality of the patient's life through a pleasurable and supportive group experience.

For caring staff and caring persons. The groups are meant (1) to demonstrate, to relatives, caring persons, and staff, methods for suitable communication with their patients and relatives and ways of helping and working with them, thereby easing some of the emotional difficulties in giving care. Characteristically, caring relatives are faced with the tragedy of watching their loved ones gradually lose their cognitive and physical capacities. Personality changes occur in the patient, and behavior may be erratic and difficult, sometimes even abusive and assaultive. The family feels keenly both the physical and the emotional strains of caring (NIMH, 1984). Similarly, caring staff in the institution need both information and support. Although often they cannot participate in the group, because of work pressures, they are welcome to attend whenever they can. In addition, videotaped sessions (authorized by the family and patients themselves) have been used in in-service programs to augment staff understanding of the patients and of the group process (Saul and Saul, 1983). Other goals are (2) to impart to caring persons a better understanding of the cause and course of the illness and to teach techniques they may use in their daily interactions with patients; (3) to expand understanding of individual patients through observation of their functioning at the highest possible level in the group with their peers; (4) to impart information about nursing home placement and to discuss factors to be considered when placement becomes an issue; and (5) to provide family caregivers (a) supportive intervention to counter feelings of hopelessness, helplessness, and aloneness, and (b) some respite from responsibility through the immediate experience of the group.

Some months after the outpatient group was initiated, a most dramatic incident occurred.

From the very first meeting, the group had seated itself in two concentric semicircles—patients in the inner circle, caring persons in the outer circle. One cold Wednesday morning—this was about the twelfth session—only seven of the ten patients and their caregivers were able to attend. When the therapist and the group settled down, it was noted with some surprise that they had formed but a single semicircle. Mr. C. (a caregiver) explained, saying, "We'd like to join the inner circle, Dr. Saul. You see, this is therapy for us as well." In that moment one of the therapist's hitherto unshared goals for the group was realized, as Mr. C. went on to describe how important the group was for all of them!

As an aid in diagnosis. Diagnosis of Alzheimer's Disease is particularly difficult and is definite only after a brain autopsy. For a living patient the diagnosis is considered presumptive, as there are not "as yet adequate definite diagnostic techniques for the living" (Heston and White, 1983).

Diagnosis of the living patient is made chiefly through elimination of other possibilities, through analysis of a carefully elicited history, and through observation of symptoms. Because of this, close observation over a period of time (as in the group setting) becomes an additional, reliable dimension of the diagnostic process. Observation of the patient's behavior and response to stimulation and motivation may corroborate or raise questions about the accuracy of the diagnosis. The individual's participation in group activity reveals, to the trained clinician, a reliable picture of the person's cognitive losses. Such observation over time assists in assessing whether memory loss is deepening or memory improving, and whether or not there is continuing deterioration.

Criteria for Group Membership

The criteria for selecting members for the group are flexible and general. Any demented patient who can relate to the therapist and/or the patients within the group setting is accepted. A second general criterion is the patient's willingness and capacity to participate (after engaging in an intake interview with the therapists).

The only persons not accepted into the group are those whose behavior would so disrupt the group that it could not function—e.g., loud, perseverant, or agitated behavior which is uncontrollable in the group. Even such a person might be accepted at some later date, when the group has settled into a "culture" into which one agitated or acting-out person might be introduced. Such a person might be calmed for an hour of group participation at some acceptable level.

If there is any doubt, and the patient is willing, a trial period may be attempted. It is also made clear to all group members that attendance is completely voluntary.

Both groups were led by coleaders: a trained group therapist and a cotherapist trainee (in the institution the latter was the unit social worker; in the community, a graduate social work student).

Referral and Intake

Patients were referred in keeping with designated criteria, which were the same for both groups. The intake process involved a review of patient history and medical condition as well as an interview with each patient.

In the community, in addition to the neurological examination, intake included a careful history taking. This involved the patient as much as possible, but also the caring person. The latter was included (1) because a good additional informant is usually needed, and (2) because this person was also to be a group member.

In the institution, referral to the group is made by the interdisciplinary health care team, which develops an individualized care plan for each patient. History and background are obtained from the patient's chart.

The interviews consisted of conversations with each patient (appropriately different for each) designed to evaluate mental status and level of orientation; evaluate ability to communicate and participate in a group; evaluate short- and long-term memory; describe the purpose and nature of the group to each patient; and invite the person to attend. Intake interviews are conducted with careful attention to the general criteria, and to the appropriateness of the group modality for each individual. This process initiates the therapeutic relationship between therapist and member (patient or caregiver) and sets the first phase of the group "contact."

GROUP PLAN, PROCESS, AND EVALUATION

Before each meeting, the cotherapists conduct a "preview"—a brief planning session to anticipate needs of the group and of individuals that might have developed since the last meeting. Flexible plans for the content of the meeting are finalized at this point. After each meeting the leaders conduct a group "review" to assess the process, members' participation, and progress, to identify the needs which may have emerged during the session, and to plan follow-up during the week or for the next session.

An additional dimension of the evaluation process involves the group members themselves. At various points in the life of both groups, members are asked to evaluate the group experience, responding to such questions as, What did we accomplish today? Was this a good group? What do you think happened in the group today?

These questions are routinely introduced toward the close of a session, as they also help the patients recapitulate their experience of the hour. Some interesting responses from the record reveal the members' feelings and ability to evaluate the group.

After a problem-solving session, Mr. B. (a patient) said, "It's teamwork. We went slow and slow and slow and then we got there!"

After a discussion about early memories, and some tears, the members were asked if they approved of such a discussion. The patients' replies included: "It makes me feel better to remember my mother and father." "Yes, it is sad to think they are dead, but I like to talk about them."

A final question is often, "What shall we do next week?" Members sometimes suggest reading the newspaper or a story, or singing a song. One responded, "Just talking like we did today would be all right too!"

Such comments help to guide the leaders in their planning. More important, they are evaluative feedback, confirming the group in its purposes. An important evaluative note in the two groups discussed here was the perfect attendance of members in both groups, exceptions being made only for illness and, in the community group, very inclement weather. Even when members expressed negative feelings about participating (and this did occur), they still came the following week.

Like any other group, the group "culture" developed over a period of time. In their beginning phase, the groups required the most active motivation by the leaders (Yalom, 1975). Then, after several sessions, six or seven members began to respond with greater initiative. By the tenth session, almost every group member had shown some level of response in the interaction, sometimes even initiating discussion or activity.

Group leaders come prepared for each session, knowing that content will vary each time, depending on the needs and concerns of group members. The group leaders are flexible and try to help members take the initiative in suggesting the content of the meeting.

At the very first session, the basic "contract" is drawn up with the members—that is, the purposes and expectations for the group are explained. Basically they are described as the opportunity to have an interesting social experience and discuss matters of mutual concern. In addition, we tell them, "We will help you think." These points are repeated at various points in the group's life, and members are reminded of them, especially after significant incidents and discussions.

From the very first session, some structure is introduced into the flow of the group meeting. In both groups the "name exercise" has proven to be an excellent way to begin the sessions. The therapist introduces himself first and then the person on his right and on his left. The next person is asked to do the same thing, and so on around the circle. In the beginning especially (but for many, at all meetings), group members did not recall one another's names. The leader would suggest in such instances that the person ask the next one's name. This exercise serves several purposes. Using one's name is, of course, a basic means of identification for self and others. For the confused person, such affirmation helps self-confirmation, and confirms the reality of the moment. The game is also an exercise in telling right from left (many patients could), as well as in recalling one's own name, and the names of others (many could not).

Of even greater importance, however, the game provides a means of "instant socialization," interaction, hand-shaking, and eye contact, all of which are important in the identification and socialization process. In both groups there was much humor, in both remembering and not remembering names. There were also instances in which people made supportive and encouraging comments: "I don't know her name, but I do remember her beautiful face," or "How could I forget such a kind-looking person?"

Very often, members who clasped hands during the introduction continued to hold hands for a while afterward, or to relate to each other through eye contact, smiles, and body language.

These are the real values of this exercise, as it is not expected that people will actually remember the names. In the nursing home group, the group members all lived on the same unit, all ate together, met in other group activities, and saw the unit social worker every single day. Yet for the most part they did not remember her name or each other's. Nevertheless, there was a special bonding within the group that carried over to warm hugs and greetings all week long. Even though *names* were not remembered, *people* were. After the name exercise, discussions or activities were initiated, either by therapists or by group members. The sessions generally closed with some evaluative discussion and some planning for the next meeting. Some highlights from group records illustrate the group's process, concerns, and uses.

Bathing

As soon as the session began, the therapist noted the sadness in Mrs. K.'s face. (Mrs. K., eighty-two, is caring for her husband, Mr.

K., who is eighty-four.) "What happened?" he asked her. She began
to describe how difficult it has become to bathe Mr. K. and to get him
to change his underwear. "He was always such a clean man! Showered
and changed every day! Now when I ask him to cooperate he becomes
angry and raises his hand to me. We've been married sixty years, and
he never raised a hand to me. What can I do? Can you help me?"

When the therapist asked Mr. K. to respond, he smiled sweetly
and said, "I bathe, I change my clothes, no problem!" The other
caring persons were involved in the discussion. Various ideas were
exchanged including that of hiring a male aide to help bathe Mr. K.
Patients, too, were drawn into the discussion. Mr. G. (a patient) attempted to reason with Mr. K., who insisted again there was no problem. Mr. G. said to the therapist, "Dr. Saul, he just doesn't remember."
At this point the therapist suggested that further discussion might
embarrass Mr. K. and that perhaps now he will be more cooperative.
Mrs. K. leaned over and held Mr. K.'s hand. At the next session she
reported that she had hired a male aide and that Mr. K. had been
more cooperative. In this instance, the therapist's response to a nonverbal message touched off an important event in the group.

Personal hygiene is a frequent problem, as is a patient's abusive
and angry behavior. The discussion in the group related to both
intellectual and emotional concerns. When the male aide was suggested, Mrs. K. was advised that an Alzheimer's patient may not recognize his own wife, and Mr. K. may have been seeing her as a totally
strange female before whom he did not want to undress. This idea
also mitigated her dismay over his assaultive gesture. Support was
given to Mrs. K. by her caring peers and also by the other patients.
The presence of Mr. K. made it possible for her to release the tensions
on the spot by holding his hand. Such discussions are emotionally
healing as well as problem-solving. The presence and limited involvement of the patients make the discussions even more poignant and
relieves some of the pressure.

Death

Mr. Z. (who was being cared for by his brother) had died since
the last meeting. Death was by asphyxiation, just after a meal. The
patients expressed their dismay by repeating, "He died! He died!"
(even though they did not recall Mr. Z.). The caring persons decided
to contact Mr. Z.'s brother. The therapist, wishing to have a more
profound exploration of feelings, turned to Mr. C. (a caregiver) and

asked him directly how he felt about the death. Mr. C. thoughtfully replied, "About our feelings—how we would feel if it happened. I guess I'd feel guilty. Why couldn't I help my wife?" Mrs. A. (another caregiver) asked, "How could such a thing happen? How could he just choke to death?" Others began to share their feelings of fright, doubt, and guilt—and to talk more freely.

After a while, the therapist reminded them about the course of Alzheimer's disease and the decrease of brain-muscle communication, a condition that may result in incontinence, choking, etc. Mr. Z.'s death, then, was not the result of poor care or inadequate attention, but of the progress of the illness. The medical examiner's report was "death by asphyxiation caused by Alzheimer's disease." It was decided that we invite a medical doctor to the next session to discuss some of these facts.

This important discussion, initiated by the therapist, dealt with significant concerns. Feelings were freely shared. During the discussion, patients also expressed their concerns. Mr. A. (a patient in the early stage of the illness) turned to his wife and said, "You see, dear, you can't be responsible for what this sickness may do to me!"

Sex

Mrs. S. (age sixty-three) came into the group flushed and upset. She takes care of her husband, Mr. S., age sixty-six. As soon as the group began she said, "Maybe I'm out of order, Dr. Saul, but I must talk to you all. I need help. My husband approached me sexually last night and I couldn't stand it! He refused to give up and I finally gave in, but I feel as if I'd been raped!"

She began to cry, and was comforted by caring persons and patients alike. Mr. C. (a caregiver in his sixties) said, "Maybe it's because I'm a man, but sex is the one area in which my wife seems to remember. She often approaches me for affection and touching. I find this is one time we communicate very well. What do you think, Dr. Saul?"

The therapist turned to the group, noted a tear in Mr. S.'s eye, and asked him directly whether the discussion was painful to him. "No," said Mr. S., "I really try hard but—" And he stopped. It was clear he had lost the subject. Mrs. S. leaned over to him and put her arm around him. He kissed her hand.

Mr. A. (a patient in the early stages) said, "Maybe if you give him more open affection he won't be so aggressive and demanding." Mrs. A. then added, "Most of the time my husband is so gentle and normal, I forget he is ill."

The therapist then took the opportunity to suggest that different couples have different styles, and that there are differences in attitudes about sex, as about anything else. The group agreed that they find this kind of discussion helpful and would talk about it again when appropriate.

For Mrs. S. there was clear therapeutic value in this opportunity to share her feelings. The feedback was nonjudgmental, nonthreatening, and helpful. The comments of the others indicated to Mrs. S. that sexual communication might still be an open avenue if allowed, and might ease tensions in other areas.

For both patients and caregivers, this supportive discussion was accompanied by hand-holding among couples, softened looks on anxious faces, and a generally tender atmosphere.

Problem Solving

In our review after the last session, we decided to plan a problem-solving session. We brought a mango to the group. The exercise was to identify the fruit and where it came from.

After our usual warm-up, the fruit was introduced. Two mangos were passed around for feeling, smelling, weighing, etc. The leaders asked leading questions: What does it look like? How does it feel? Where does it grow? Each answer was used to evoke another. Clues were given and as the group became more and more excited (twenty minutes later) they were asked what was happening. Answers came such as, "We are working together," and "We are using teamwork to get answers." The fruit had been described as an orange, or grapefruit, as heavy, as a favorite fruit. Finally through repeated questions it was determined that it grew in places like Hawaii, Florida, Cuba, California, and Puerto Rico. Mr. A. very proudly stated, "You see we work together to get answers. It takes two to tango!" The therapist held up the fruit and said, "Is this a tango?" "No," answered Mrs. C., "it's a mango!" The group cheered her for her answer and she responded, "Anyone knows it's a mango!"

The pleasure, excitement, joy, and pride at this session was indescribable. It seemed to the group and the therapists that all purposes had been fulfilled at one time. Cognitive efforts were accompanied by the emotional pleasure and esteem resulting from achievement.

The session ended with everyone eating pieces of the mango, discussing the taste, wiping up the juice and helping one another. What fun, what accomplishment!

OUTCOMES

Some outcomes of these group sessions have been identified by therapists, caregivers (relatives as well as staff), and patients, and have been recognized by administrators in the two settings.

Modification of patient behavior. This was reported by family members, as well as by staff in the institution. The chief of maintenance, for example, viewing the tapes in in-service, commented to the staff that prior to the group experience Mr. B. had urinated habitually on the radiator in his room, but has since stopped. Nurses and aides commented on the fact that it was now easier to communicate with some of the patients and to give them care.

Improved socialization among group members. Even though they did not remember intellectually, there was an emotional bond among group members and with staff, especially in the institution.

Improved methods of caregiving. New techniques, suggested in the group, were attempted, and both family and staff reported back to the group appropriately.

Emotional and psychological support to families and patients. Opportunity was provided to express real feelings in appropriate ways.

Existential experiences. Thinking, recalling, enjoying the moment, using judgment, and reasoning were experienced as possible.

A word about humor and its helpfulness in the group: The pervasive depression and hopelessness which characterizes the suffering of these patients and their caregivers is a natural area for the gentle and appropriate use of humor. The group members (patients and others) were encouraged to laugh, to see humor in some situations, and to tell jokes. The atmosphere of gloom in the early sessions (very clearly noted in both written and videotaped records of the meetings) was replaced by a more helpful and also a more cheerful atmosphere in later sessions. The group itself is an alleviating experience. The infusion of humor, along with other helping techniques, is an important therapeutic dimension.

These outcomes were clearly perceived and verbalized, to the point where both settings are actively considering extending the programs. In the mental health center it has been recommended that a day hospital program (five days a week)* for these patients be developed with the involvement of family members (Mace, 1984). In the

---

*The five day a week program was successfully implemented in January of 1986. It was an immediate and continuing success.

institution, such therapy groups for patients and their caregivers are an important component of the total treatment plan and should be built appropriately into program offerings.

REFERENCES

HCOA (1983), Drug use and misuse: A growing concern for older Americans. Joint Hearing—Select Committee on Aging. Publication 98–392. Washington, D.C.: U.S. Government Printing Office.

Heston, L. L., & White. J. A. (1983), *Dementia: A Practical Guide to Alzheimer's Disease and Related Illnesses*. New York: Freeman.

Mace, N. (1984), Day care for demented clients. *Hospital & Community Psychiat.*, 10:979–981.

——— Rabens, P. V. (1981), *The Thirty-Six Hour Day*. Baltimore: Johns Hopkins University Press.

National Institute on Aging (1980), Age Page: Senility, Myth or Madness. National Institutes of Health.

NIMH (1984), Progress report on Alzheimer's disease. Publication 84–2500, Vol. II. Washington, D.C.: U.S. Government Printing Office.

Reisberg, B. (1981), *Brain Failure*. New York: The Free Press.

——— (1982), Office management and treatment of primary degenerative dementia. In *Psychiatric Annals* 12:631–637.

Saul, S. R., & Saul, S. (1983), "We'll Help You Think" videotape series: Herbert H. Lehman College & Kingsbridge Heights Nursing Home 1983.

Trubo, R. (1984), The growing problem of Alzheimer's disease. *Medical World News for Psychiatrists*, Sept. 13, pp. 24–34.

Yalom, I. D. (1975), *The Theory and Practice of Group Psychotherapy*. New York: Basic Books.

Part V
*The Arts in
Group Therapy*

16

The Arts as Psychotherapeutic Modalities with Groups of Older People

SHURA SAUL, Ed.D., A.C.S.W.

The arts are an essential and integral part of our humanness, and through them we are each and all of us put closely in touch with our universe. The capacity to create and experience music, poetry, art, dance, and drama is inherent within each individual as well as within the human collective. Indeed, the arts are built into the very anatomy of the human body, which itself mirrors, parallels, and combines the artistic activities and movements of the universe. As creatures of life, we are each part of the rhythms of time and tides, the music of water and wind, the beauties of earth and sky, and the eternal drama of struggle, search, and survival. The human quest is a combination of intellect and emotion through which the arts are threaded as unifying bonds toward understanding, enlightenment, expression, and communication.

Creativity and artistic experience, as integral facets of the human personality, have been considered by the philosophers and thinkers concerned with understanding human behavior. As Jung (1920) wrote, "Psychology and *aesthetics* will always have to turn to one another for help, and the one will not invalidate the other" (p. 87).

Psychotherapy seeks to help the personality improve its inner balance so that a person may live and function on a more appropriate and reality-oriented level, and to assist in developing improved social functioning toward the enjoyment of a healthier, more satisfying existence. The practitioner must address the inner personality needs of the person seeking help; must examine the particular life or crises which have impelled the seeking of help; and must help the individual

to develop insight, to change, and to improve relationships in both
inner and outer worlds. This process is as true for elderly persons as
for those of any age.

Cath's concept of omniconvergence (1965) holds that for older
people a convergence of many life factors and problems within a
relatively short period of time characterizes and complicates the aging
process, often making it a very difficult time of life—painful and
sometimes overwhelming. Psychotherapy can help some older people
cope better with this convergence of problems. Ingebretzen (1977)
summarizes four main areas of problems encountered among elderly
patients, areas not mutually exclusive:

> *organic brain syndrome*—which can bring about psychotic condi-
> tions; *problems the individual has had from earlier years,* such as neu-
> rotic symptoms and character disorders; *special crises* which arise
> frequently in the later years and represent a break with continuity
> of earlier life (retirement, death of spouse or friends, isolation,
> illness); *existential tasks* the elderly have in integrating their earlier
> life with present life circumstances, the acceptance of death and
> seeking meaning in their lives. [p. 322]

These categorize the substantive life issues with which older persons must grapple. Psychotherapy offers possibilities for alleviating
the emotional suffering they inflict. In this process the creative arts
can be extremely helpful, especially where efforts are directed toward
regenerating health through the reawakening of an individual's in-
nately human capacities.

Elderly persons, like any age group, are not a homogeneous population. Like any other person in psychotherapy, an older person
must be assessed for individual needs and appropriate treatment
methods. Treatment through experience with one or more of the arts
is useful for some people—perhaps for more than is currently be-
lieved. The arts by their very nature are expressive of feelings and
are media of communication, both intrapsychic and social. Despite
their obvious modal differences, this characteristic is common to all
of them. The very differences among the modalities themselves expand the range of possibilities for the necessary individualization of
treatment. The arts offer a spectrum of media utilizing sound, sights,
and words, as well as abstract symbols and fantasy. Because of their
profound integrity with the essence of the human condition, the arts
should be viewed not as "nonverbal modalities" (a negative concept)

but rather as "supraverbal"—that is, "beyond-the-verbal." That is, each art form has its unique communicative facet that bypasses words or even the need for words. Each presents intellectual and emotional ideas eliciting responses that may not require words. Human communication should not be viewed as either "verbal" or "nonverbal"; the very positing of this dichotomy falsely suggests that language is the single primary medium of human communication.

Susanne Langer notes (1957):

> The most astounding and developed symbolic device humanity has evolved is language. By means of language we can conceive the intangible, incorporeal things we call our ideas, and the equally inostensible elements of our perceptual world we call facts . . . this use of language is discourse; . . . it is a highly versatile, amazingly powerful pattern . . . [p. 21] there is a great deal of experience that is knowable, . . . yet defies discursive formulation [p. 22] . . . Whatever resists projection into the discursive form of language is indeed hard to hold in conception and perhaps impossible to communicate, in the proper and strict sense of the word "communicate." But fortunately our logical intuition, or form-perception, is really more powerful than we commonly believe, and our knowledge — genuine knowledge, understanding — is considerably wider than our discourse. [p. 23]

Discursive language does not readily express emotional life. Works of art do. These ideas are important to the psychotherapist, for they suggest the creative arts as powerful vehicles through which feelings may be expressed, shared, and reexamined. Experiences recapitulated under circumstances different from their origins may be "re-felt" in new ways. The arts are powerful vehicles, also, through which earlier, hurtful misconceptions, relived emotionally, may be reshaped, possibly becoming more understandable and less hurtful. They are vehicles through which we can discover and rediscover ourselves and others who are important to us. Thus, artistic experiences may be powerful vehicles through which trauma and injury to the personality may be treated. In short, the artistic experience may be used as a healing modality.

Langer notes further that

> a work of art presents feeling . . . for our contemplation, making it visible or audible in some way perceived through a symbol, not

inferable from a symptom. Artistic form is congruent with the dynamic forms of our direct, sensuous, mental and emotional life; works of art are projections of "felt life," as Henry James called it, into spatial, temporal and poetic structure. They are images of feeling that formulate it for our cognition. What is artistically good is whatever articulates and presents feeling to our understanding. [p. 25]

A therapeutic modality must be suited to the individual who is to be helped. To some frail elderly persons (as indeed to frail persons of any age) the use of words to express feelings may appear too threatening, too complex, too burdensome. The experience of an ego-compatible art form can be supportive, soothing, or motivational. It becomes an acceptable medium through which distress may be alleviated and the ego freed to a condition of decreased vulnerability and greater strength.

The older person in need of psychotherapy is often reeling from the blows and traumas that have accompanied the aging process. The changes this person faces and must master are often accompanied by a sense of depression, of hopelessness, of loss of control over one's life. When life becomes a dismal struggle threatening even survival, it may well become as colorless and passionless as it appears futureless. In addition to specific individual problems, this is often the affectual context of the life of the frail elderly person in psychotherapy.

The infinite nuances of the emotional spectrum offered by the various creative arts suggests possibilities for "beginning where the person is" emotionally, and helping him or her through to a more colorful, passionate, and future-oriented existence—even when "one small step at a time" seems the only possibility. "The creative arts," writes Zwerling (1979)

> evoke responses precisely at the level at which psychotherapists work to engage their patients, more directly and more immediately than any of the more traditional verbal therapies. . . . the nonverbal media employed by creative arts therapists more directly tap emotional rather than cognitive process in patients. . . . the creative arts therapists deal closer to primary thought processes than do verbal therapists. [p. 843]

One of the most prevalent myths about elderly persons is "that they all decline in intellectual function; that aging is a time of withdrawal and disengagement . . . that life becomes purposeless and use-less" (Butler, 1975, p. 98).

In the case of the frail elderly, outward appearances often support this misconception. The physical appearance of a frail or disabled person of any age often belies the strength, beauty, and vibrancy that pulsates within. Whether they live in their own homes or in institu-tions, many frail old people are isolated and lonely, and have retreated within themselves simply through lack of opportunity for satisfying human interaction. In the institution a person often withdraws from the communal group in an effort to preserve individuality and privacy within a threatening and difficult communal living situation. There may be a faraway look in the eye, a despondent droop of the head, a body language of rejection and withdrawal, a positioning of self away from others. Yet, on approaching such a person, one often finds greater responsiveness than the outward appearance and accompa-nying stereotype suggest. For the most part, the isolated, frail, disabled person hungers for the normalcy of human contact, for the oppor-tunity to communicate on one's own level with another person, to express oneself somehow.

However, some elderly people have undergone such traumatic losses and changes in their inner and outer worlds that they may not respond readily to customary everyday overtures. They may require more aggressive motivation, more skilled intervention into their iso-lation, before they respond.

The creative arts offer ways to reach beyond this apathy and withdrawal, to present an array of "feeling experiences" to tempt the emotional and intellectual palate. An experience with the arts fulfills the spirit without necessarily demanding a return. Yet for many peo-ple the artistic experience does ultimately elicit a response—first within the emotions of the individual, then at some level of inner cognition, and finally in interaction with the person's external world.

Two very old, very physically ill nursing home patients, de-pressed, agitated, and both wheelchair bound, began to paint and draw for the very first time. "It gives me a feeling of accomplishment. I look at my picture when it is finished and I say to myself, 'I really did this. I really did!'" The other, deeply deformed by arthritis, said softly, "It eases the pain."

Along with other stereotypes, old people are thought to have lost their "creative juices." However, this too is a misconception. In fact, a review of the artistic world reveals the many geniuses who have continued to create, and to grow in their capacity to create, through the eighth and ninth decades of life. On a less grandiose scale, we have seen many older people develop new interests and participate in artistic endeavors as soon as opportunities for such activity have presented themselves. In fact, for some, the later years may offer new dimensions of creativity. "Increased age," writes Taylor (1975), "does not necessarily produce decreased creativity. We have found several indications that certain types of creativity reduce at certain times during the life span, but during advanced age much of this creativity can be recaptured" (p. 113).

Taylor suggests five dispositions to creativity. The earliest type he calls *"expressive spontaneity* found in the spontaneous drawings of children, extemporaneous dance, . . . etc." *Technical proficiency* is a second form which develops out of the first. Then, from adolescence through the early twenties, comes *inventive ingenuity*, which takes the form of idealized drawings, etc. During the later twenties and thirties comes *innovative flexibility*. "A final form of creativity," he writes, "has its roots in *emergentive creativity* or the disposition to create original or essentially new ideas . . . [It is] largely ideational and seems to flourish in the late fifties and sixties, indeed for some many people into their 80's and 90's." The implications of these concepts and of supportive research, he concludes, "are that creativity need not necessarily decline with age, but may change its form toward a deeper and more basic form of creativity . . ." (pp. 114–116).

"I was very sick, and thought I was going to die," said one elderly Puerto Rican man to the group. "I prayed to live—and promised myself that if I would live, I would turn to painting and poetry, which I had longed to do since I was a child. But I had always had to work hard for a living, and could never follow that calling. Now, I said, if I live, I shall paint and write." He then proceeded to tell the group how he had joined a senior citizens art program and for the first time in his life found his "true self" through painting and writing.

Human beings neither live nor function in a vacuum. Even the most reclusive hermit is communicating a message through his avoidance of social contact. Slavson (1952) wrote,

> Among the most important developments in psychiatry and psychology in recent times is the recognition that man is essentially a group animal. . . . The most important value to character formation of group experience is the modification or elimination of egocentricity and psychological insularity. It increases the ability

to feel with other people . . . that is, to establish positive identi-
fications. [p. 1]

It has been suggested that we are not only gregarious animals
with a liking to be in the sight of our fellows, but that we have an
innate propensity to get ourselves noticed and noticed favorably by
our kind. Kris (1952) writes,

> Wherever artistic creation takes place, the idea of a public exists,
> though the artist may attribute this role only to one real or im-
> aginary person. . . . wherever the unconscious aspect of artistic
> creation is studied, a public of some kind emerges. . . .
> Art, . . . consciously or unconsciously, serves the purpose of com-
> munication. We distinguish two stages: one in which the artist's
> id communicates to the ego, and one in which the same intra-
> psychic processes are submitted to others. [pp. 60–61]

The artistic experience within the group framework fuses these
varied needs and processes—that is, the desire for positive identification with others, the requirement for a "showcase for favorable
notice and sharing," and the expression of the inner communication
within the personality.

A creative art experience in a group has the unique advantage
of offering a person the opportunity to conform and be different
almost at the same time, and to communicate both privately and publicly almost at the same time. This remarkable situation is true whether
the person in the group is listening, participating in, responding to,
or creating the experience.

An artistic experience is lived on so many levels at once that a
person "feels" oneself in any number of dimensions at the same time;
feels a sense of aliveness, of fullness, of creative functioning and a
general engagement with life through the medium. The arts motivate,
initiate, generate, provoke response. The person is stirred, even when
the response seems to remain secret and within. The individual must
make choices in the way in which the response will be expressed,
whether inwardly or outwardly.

The opportunity to make these choices, no matter how brief or
imperceptible, helps the person feel more in control. Because the
choice is the individual's, the group becomes a place of trust and
security.

A person's most secret response may be seen by the therapist in some almost imperceptible change—changes in the lines of the face, body stance, the fluttering of an eyelid, the thrust of an eyebrow, a light in the eyes, the nodding of a head, the waving of a finger, the flicker of a smile or frown. The therapist notes this and builds upon it through the selected medium.

A group member is encouraged to express emotion or ideas, to suggest innovation. At some time or other each individual has the opportunity to share "the limelight" (if this seems appropriate for the person), if only through a special kind of participation with fellow group members, if only to be openly recognized for his or her presence.

As in all groups, the uniqueness of each individual is accepted as an offering to guide the member and the group through a shared experience to work the individual's idea into the general flow of ideas (whether pro or con, verbal or not) and so demonstrate how each member has something to give to others, while simultaneously *living* the experience.

Differences from others is as valid an offering as any, and to be accepted as a gift to the group. The creative arts seek out differences, encourage individual expressions, and the therapist utilizes these to enhance the experience and the confidence of the person and the group.

These possibilities are especially helpful for older persons who are insecure about their capacities at a point in their lives when they are losing so much—for those older persons who feel they have lost their very "selves," as well as their capacities to cope and master current life conflicts.

Yalom (1975) suggests that "therapeutic change . . . occurs through an interplay of various guided experiences" that he calls "curative factors." He offers eleven primary categories of these, all of which readily suggest the valuable uses of the creative arts in groups for the psychotherapy of elderly persons. These factors include universality, altruism, the development of socializing techniques, imitative behavior, interpersonal learning, corrective recapitulation of the primary family group, catharsis, group cohesiveness, existential factors, the instillation of hope and imparting of knowledge (pp. 3–17).

Working through a creative experience within a group is satisfying and healthy. Following and leading, learning and teaching, listening and telling, observing and doing are all activities which offer endless possibilities for creative social interchange and improved social functioning. Participation in any group allows a person to respond with individualized timing; there is opportunity to "hold back" before "giving out." In the creative arts group, there is opportunity to participate, observe, and enjoy—to be nourished before being expected to produce or perform. Engagement with an ego-syntonic medium is itself an immediate emotional and therapeutic nurturing.

The arts offer an opportunity to express feelings in a nonthreatening way but, further, they offer an exchange of these feelings for others of beauty and power. Thus, the arts themselves have a healing quality which, within the cathartic process, gives healthy release from emotional pain—something "to feel better about." Such sharing within the group spawns feelings of trust and comradeship. This, plus the skilled and sensitive leadership of the therapist (who helps connect the total experience with personal growth), helps to center the experience within the person.

Finally, the arts themselves offer a "lift," a sense that hope may be renewed, that there is yet more in life to experience. A sense of the future pushes slowly against the lost yesterdays and the seemingly useless present. Here is something to make tomorrow more acceptable.

"The artist," says Henry Moore (1952), "works with a concentration of his whole personality and the conscious part of it resolves conflicts, organizes memories, and prevents him from trying to walk in two directions at the same time" (p. 73). To a person who may feel that all the structures of life have gotten out of hand and beyond control, concentrating on an artistic creation mobilizes healthy resources and offers a purpose for the present moment and the next one as well. A sense of mastery reassures the person who feels a loss of control in vital areas of life. This helps to ease depression and hopelessness. Butler (1975) writes,

> Among creative people, I find great pressure to be inventive and reinventive of different versions of self. It seems to me that insufficient attention has been given to the constricting effects of identity as the concept is commonly used. . . . a continuing, lifelong identity crisis is a sign of good health, and the right to have such a crisis is one of the important rights to life. Human beings need the freedom to live with change, to invent and reinvent themselves a number of times throughout their lives. [pp. 103–105]

For the older person, whose external existence has been reshaped through a series of circumstances converging within a relatively brief period of time, an identity crisis is almost an axiomatic accompaniment. The arts, as well as other media, offer innumerable ways of "reinventing" oneself, as Polansky (1975) notes:

> In my professional work I have sometimes tentatively suggested something of this creative process for older persons caught up in problems which drain their energies. I suggest to them that they try art, music or anything that has meaning for that person. . . . I tell people not only to try looking at art or listening to music but making it . . . creating it. . . .[p. 111]

Artistic creativity offers a way of filling some of the voids created by the numerous losses experienced in the aging process. They are neither substitutes nor stopgaps but meaningful life experiences in themselves offering color, passion, and pleasure, stirring the imagination and motivating initiative. Not all of us can be Leonardos, Beethovens, or even Grandma Moseses, but for many elderly persons the combination of arts and group modality helps, treats, and heals—all goals of the therapeutic process.

Zwerling (1979) writes, "Those who organize programs to treat people rather than to cure disease will find creative arts therapies invaluable" (p. 844). We might add: for helping elderly people in groups.

REFERENCES

Butler, R. N. (1975), The creative life and old age. In: *Successful Aging: A Conference Report*, ed. E. Pfeiffer. Durham, N.C.: Duke University Press, pp. 97–109.
Cath, S. H. (1965), Some dynamics of the middle and later years. In: *Crisis Intervention*, ed. H. Parad. New York: Family Service Association of America, pp. 174–192.
Ingebretzen, R. (1977), Psychotherapy and the elderly. *Psychotherapy: Theory, Research & Practice*, 14:319–333.
Jung, C. G. (1920), The spirit of man in art and literature. In: *The Collected Works of C. G. Jung, Vol. 15: Psychology and Literature*. New York: Pantheon, 1966, pp. 84–105.
Kris, E. (1952), *Psychoanalytic Explorations in Art*. New York: International Universities Press.
Langer, S. K. (1957), Expressiveness. In: *Problems of Art*. New York: Scribners, pp. 13–26.
Moore, H. (1952), Notes on sculpture. In: *The Creative Process*, ed. B. Ghiselin. New York: Mentor, pp. 73–78.

Polansky, G. (1975), Age and creativity. In: *Successful Aging: A Conference Report,* ed. E. Pfeiffer. Durham, N.C.: Duke University Press, pp. 109–113.

Slavson, S. R. (1952), *An Introduction to Group Therapy.* New York: International Universities Press.

Taylor, I. A. (1975), Patterns of creativity and aging. In: *Successful Aging: A Conference Report,* ed. E. Pfeiffer. Durham, N.C.: Duke University Press, pp. 113–118.

Yalom, I. D. (1975), *The Theory and Practice of Group Psychotherapy.* New York: Basic Books.

Zwerling, I. (1979), The creative arts therapies as real therapies. *Hospital & Community Psychiat.,* 3:841–844.

17

The Poetry Group

SHURA SAUL, Ed.D., A.C.S.W.

Feeling comes from the soul
Words come from the mind.
This makes a terrible difference.

In this brief verse Mrs. A.H. expressed what poetry means to
her. Poetry has the unique distinction of combining both verbal and
nonverbal artistry, as music and imagery are integral to poetic expression. They are, in fact, among the basic ingredients of poetry and
distinguish it as an art form from other kinds of verbal expression.

Within the institution, opportunities for self-expression are severely limited. Depersonalization is a common characteristic of its
residents (Gossett, 1968), because of the very nature of institutional
organization (Goffman, 1961). One of the most serious threats to the
individual resident in a long-term care facility is a loss of identity, the
struggle for which is a lifetime activity for each person, young or old,
sick or well. For the elderly resident in long-term care, the struggle
is intensified by the circumstances of illness and dependency, feelings
of rejection and abandonment. It is further exacerbated by the general
pervasive atmosphere of illness (mental and physical) and the perspective of long-term residency within the institution.

For the caring staff and the institution as a whole, there is the
ever present challenge and pressing need to try to organize life's
routines and activities so as to maximize individual expression. One
way to do this is to develop small groups for those individuals who
can find themselves and each other best in a small organized situation
carved within the larger, more amorphous one (Scheidlinger, 1980).

This was one of the motivations for developing the poetry group at Kingsbridge Heights Manor. It was open to any resident interested in listening to, reading, and discussing poetry. In addition, it was hoped that some poetry would be written by the group members.

Eleven women came to the first meeting. (Others began to participate at a later point.) They were all known to the group therapist and to each other. The ladies included Mrs. H.W., a quiet, cultured woman well-liked and respected by staff and residents alike; Mrs. F.G. and Mrs. L.V., both active in many group activities; Mrs. S.F., a deeply depressed alert and intelligent woman; Mrs. M.G., a quiet, gentle person; Mrs. L.K., a small, soft-spoken Russian lady; the charming Mrs. S.N., who is very disoriented but intelligent, lively, and kind; and Mrs. E.N., an attractive and talented new resident. A surprise member was Miss A.B., whose group participation had always been limited to mass activities like Bingo, and whose interest in poetry was most unexpected. All of these women are in their middle and late eighties, except for Mrs. H.W., who is past ninety, and Mrs. F.G. and Mrs. L.V., who are in their middle sixties.

Into the room that first meeting came two more women. The first was Mrs. J.P., a slight, dark-haired woman with an extraordinary talent for conflict with staff and residents. When she entered the room there was a perceptible and pervasive response of hostility. She was clearly persona non grata.

There was even greater disgruntlement, quite audible, when Mrs. A.H. came in. This woman is a deeply agitated, depressed resident given to acting out. She speaks in broken English with a strong Slavic accent, and her manner is simultaneously obsequious and belligerent.

The medical charts of these eleven women bear individual diagnoses that include depression, manic-depressive illness, agitation, paranoia, disorientation, and confusion. Indeed, on a day-to-day basis these individuals exhibit behavior characteristic of these conditions. It was one of the goals of this group to offer an artistic experience with poetry that might mitigate some of the symptoms and elicit healthier and more satisfying behavior.

Members and therapist arrive each week with the expectation of spending an hour together—an hour during which they share from a grab bag of thoughts and feelings and pour them through a poetic funnel into some sort of emotional, imagistic, verbal communication. Sometimes the session is begun by a member's reading aloud a poem she has written in solitude. It may begin with a question or comment by a group member, sometimes an angry comment about an incident that may have occurred earlier or elsewhere. It may begin with a discussion of a holiday or change of season, an event in the facility, or a more global incident in the news. Sometimes the therapist reads a poem, but this is usually reserved as a final alternative, as it is preferable that a group member initiate the discussion. The therapist arrives each week with a bag full of poetry books. Sometimes not a single poem is read; sometimes the hour is spent reading several. This is a freewheeling experience which grows from the needs and concerns of the members. However the group may begin, it soon settles into a discussion of material that somehow touches everyone. It has become clear over time that despite the fact that they meet within the institution, their information is shared outside the group only when permission is explicitly granted by the members. The group feels very free and members complain openly, knowing that their need for this opportunity is respected and that the content remains confidential. At one session, for example, one of the members reported an unpleasant incident with a nurse. The others began to talk about how some, though not all, of the nurses behave toward them. They then composed two pages of prose in which they set forth their ideas, as a group, about how nurses should act toward patients. This dignified piece of writing reveals how each group member sought to express her highest level of thinking about a matter that affects their daily life.

This session was difficult. Tears were shed as the women made clear their feelings of dependency upon the strangers caring for them, strangers who do not perceive them for the individuals they are, but only as patients.

After this particularly distressing session, the following poem was written by Mrs. A.H., who had emerged, through time, as a true poet. At first her image of angry behavior followed her into the group. She responded to poetry readings with emotional outbursts which, though appropriate, were greeted with stony silence by the other group members. It became clear, however, that Mrs. A.H. perceives life through an emotional spectrum of creative tensions that haunt all artists—and her modality is poetry. Even though English is not her native tongue, she manages to convey within her brief verses a universality of feeling to which the group members could all ultimately relate. Within a few months the group had learned to listen to her ideas and expression. They dropped their feelings of annoyance and impatience and realized instead that she was creating poetry that touched them in im-

portant ways. They listened appreciatively as she composed the
following poem:

To Complain

To complain
Through talking

If we have a chance
Only to talk . . .

What does it mean?
Something hurts

Very seldom is there a chance
For people to listen

If people only listened more
We would never need a psychiatrist!

In the discussion that followed, others began to express their
feelings. The discussion ended with the following lines contributed
by the women in turn as they summarized their feelings poetically.

Tears

I think the good Lord created tears
To make our hearts easier.

After a good cry
You feel much better

It relieves you.
It doesn't help?

Well, you have to cry harder.
You have to try harder.

When this verse was read back to them, the women felt that it
was indeed an authentic reflection of their feelings. The session ended

with a sense that we had shared an important hour and had together created a poem that could be shared with people outside the group. Harrower (1972) writes, "One of the prerequisites of true poetry . . . is that it transcend the immediate circumstances of its creation and becomes universal in its application" (p. 5).

Just as Mrs. A.H. became accepted in the group for her poetry and insights, so too Mrs. J.P.'s image in the group changed as she revealed herself, often through reminiscence poetry. The group shared her memories when she read:

Drawing on My Bank of Memories

It is Saturday morning and I am fanning the embers
To a flaming glow—the coal stove, windows, floor, I remember
After polishing, scrubbing and shining . . . our reward?
To the free Public Library with anticipation we headed toward
Treasures unfolding, Bible stories, Aesop's fables
Andersen's fairy tales, other lore
Sinbad, Aladdin (only two books each, but we were four!)
Homeward with magical, untold wealth
Eight books our store
Of once upon a time, and still reverberating
With enthrallment of yore!

It soon became clear that Mrs. J.P.'s agitation stemmed, at least in part, from a lifelong repression of her many artistic talents as she had lived as a "put-down" housewife and mother in a male-dominated culture and household. The women identified wholeheartedly with her when she read them the following:

As an urban and suburban woman
I have been on the firing line and
Also behind the eight ball some of the time.
Life experience has taught me not to look back
But to run with what I have, not to lack energy
Enthusiasm, mobility, vitality, alone but never lonely
To take the best and leave the rest
The whole wide world to enjoy with zest
With time running out, there is none to waste

Through sharing her poems, which she wrote in her room and then read to the group, Mrs. J.P. became accepted for the troubled and profound woman she truly was, rather than the argumentative and hostile patient she had become in the institution (Slavson, 1943).

In general, each person in the group began to verbalize her own identity as poems were read in which poets revealed and found themselves. Edna St. Vincent Millay's poem, "Renascence" was read many times and touched off exciting responses. Two members composed the following poem:

> Poetry wakes up the soul
> And through the spirit
> The soul feels much better.
>
> Somehow the soul is sleeping
> It needs a little boosting.
>
> It has a lot to do with the world today
> If there would be more expression
> Through soul and spirit
> People would be nicer to each other.

There was a growing awareness of what the group and its members meant in terms of supportive relationships. Mrs. L.K. wrote the following:

> *What Are Friends For?*
>
> To everyone it is important to find a friend
>
> It is not easy
> In order to find a friend
> You have to try to be a friend yourself.
>
> It has to be mutual
> Like marriage, it is a two-way proposition.
>
> In order to keep a friend
> Both partners have to make concessions
> If you strive toward a relationship

You have to work for it.

The very depressed Mrs. S.F. wrote:

> When you practice how to love
> You gain others' love
> Your life is fuller
> And you become a better person.

After the group had shared some poetry by Emily Dickinson and William Blake (and other immortal poets), Mrs. A.H. wrote:

> I think
> The poets did something for our souls
> They made much better people of us
> Through their art.
> Without them, life would be very very poor
> People who read their art
> Have become much better human beings.

Several of the members have died since the group began, Mrs. J.P. among them. Each time, the group spent the session remembering the lost member, mourning her and comforting themselves and one another. Death is an ever present dimension of life in the facility. Each time, the group would read some poems by the member who had died, and sometimes also a poem by a famous poet such as Emily Dickinson or Alfred Tennyson. Thus their courage and investment in life would be renewed.

The range of subjects discussed by the group was boundless. Memories, home, family, friends, nature, philosophy, humor—all were explored through poetry and restated in their own poetic imagery. Growing old, part of the identity struggle of each member, was discussed very often. The group wrote a long poem which they decided to perform as a group reading. They gave several performances for other residents, one of which was videotaped and reviewed by the group itself. A publication of their own poems, together with the work of the art therapy group, was produced and sold (Saul, 1982).

The group members often discussed the importance of the group in their lives. When the discussion touched on the fact that this was not a poetry "class," the therapist asked, "What is the difference?"

Some of the answers reveal how true to the human spirit they regard this experience: "It's a more natural thing to be in a group." "A class is regimented and a group is a friendly get-together." Unexpectedly, Miss A.B. said, "We have equal rights in the group!" And the charming, disoriented Mrs. S.N. said, "In the group, we're one for all and all for one!"

What are the therapeutic values of this group? At other times of the week, these women are dependent patients or participants in group activities. In this group, each member takes her place within the art experience. The poetry is exciting, uplifting, creative. Whether she writes a poem or listens to someone else's, she participates in the creative activity. This enhances the quality of her daily life. Her identity is elicited and confirmed, and with it comes a restoration of pride in herself.

The group plays down disabilities, overlooks pathology, and evokes the essential humanness and health of each member. It appeals to the highest level of cognitive and emotional functioning. Members begin to see new parts of themselves and each other as they touch each other in unaccustomed ways.

True feelings are expressed, shared, and ventilated. The personality of each member is encouraged to open and grow. Social behavior has been improved as self-image and esteem is restored and enhanced. The freedom and creative atmosphere of the group becomes an antidote to the suppressive aspects of the institution (Hartford, 1980).

The group session is a high spot of the week for everyone. At parting there are hugs, kisses, handshakes, and smiles. An hour of wealth and beauty has been shared, lifting the group members from the mundane, helping them cope with some of their woes, put aside others, clarify some perceptions of their realities, adjusting life perspectives. The group experience has put a special beauty into the day.

"I'm published!" said Mrs. F.G. exultantly. "I never thought I would be. Now I am somebody!"

REFERENCES

Goffman, E. (1961), *Asylums*. New York: Doubleday Anchor.

Gossett, H. (1968), Restoring identity to socially deprived and depersonalized older people. *Bull. Institute Gerontology*, 15(supp.):3–6.

Harrower, M. (1972), *The Therapy of Poetry*. Springfield, Ill.: Thomas.

Hartford, M. E. (1980), The use of group methods for work with the aged.

In: *Handbook of Mental Health and Aging*, ed. J. E. Birren & R. B. Sloan. Englewood Cliffs, N.J.: Prentice-Hall.

Saul, S., Ed. (1982), Songs of ourselves. New York: Kingsbridge Heights Nursing Home.

Scheidlinger, S. (1980), Identification: The sense of belonging and of identity in small groups. In: *Psychoanalytic Group Dynamics*. New York: International Universities Press, pp. 213–231.

Slavson, S. R. (1943), *An Introduction to Group Therapy*. New York: International Universities Press.

18

Dance Therapy Groups for the Elderly

SONYA SAMBERG, G.D.T.

THE HEALING EFFECTS OF MOVEMENT

Dance therapy is coming into its own as a valuable form of healing, for all age groups. As a form of treatment it provides the elderly a source of activity for which their hearts and souls cry out.

In every culture, rhythmic and symbolic movement has provided expression for people's fears and joys. In primitive societies today, people still communicate with the supernatural via motion to heal physical ills and to attain spiritual comfort, as an integral part of their cultural life. In modern society we tend to regard dance as a recreational activity and overlook its therapeutic qualities, its wondrous medicinal effect on the minds and bodies of the aged. "Dance," writes Kedzie Penfield (1978), "is the art form of expression through movement . . . of man's inner life. . . . movement rivals words in the completeness of the way it can express feelings. . . . no words can compare to the directness of a clenched fist or the postural collapse of an individual overcome by despair."

We are aware that mothers commonly rock their children back and forth to comfort them when they are afraid or in pain. Rhythmic processions are accompanied by stylized movements; traditional music is evoked as a catharsis in religious events, celebrations, and mourning; and many gestures accompany speech for a more easily understood concept of what is being communicated.

Important as they are, words are only symbols and require abstract thinking. Basic emotions such as hate, love, anger, and fear are first expressed in bodily change. There is no separation of mind and body; one interacts with the other; one can *change* the other. Unhappy thoughts may disturb the body's natural functioning and affect the immune system. So, too, lack of movement causes inertia, lack of exercise then bringing about depression and accompanying anxiety.

DANCE THERAPY TODAY

Dance therapy uses the healing qualities of movement and has been developed as a tool for defining and directing individual progress toward well-being—loosely defined as a sense of comfort, adjustment, and fulfillment. It has become an independent form of nonverbal therapy.

In the book *Therapeutic Dance Movement* (Caplow-Lindner, Harpaz, and Samberg, 1979), dance therapy is defined as "the use of rhythmic movement as a means of self-expression and communication that aids in the healthy integration of mind and body" (p. 37). It provides the doctor, the nurse, the instructor, or anyone else on the scene with insight into the personality of the individual and serves as an outlet for expression and socialization.

Dance therapy, as we know and use it today, began at about the end of the Second World War, during which period therapists were exploring methods of nonverbal treatment for mentally ill patients who were, more often than not, heavily medicated and unable to participate in the more traditional forms of treatment.

This new interest of therapists in nonverbal communication was shared by dancers, and it is not coincidental that a pioneer of dance therapy was both a dancer and a therapist. Marian Chace (1975), considered the nation's first dance therapist and founder of the field, practiced at St. Elizabeth Hospital in Washington, D.C. for over two decades. She explored the healing benefits of motion in a clinical context, utilizing the improvisational self-expression process of modern dance as an adjunct to psychotherapy. Her work provided therapeutic experiences involving group interaction, individual expressions, and heightened body awareness for the participants. Overlooked, then, was the tremendous impact of dance to instill in patients the important feeling of contact, self-esteem, and revitalization of self-worth. Yet many facets of these healthy attributes were regained by many elderly patients undergoing dance therapy. Thus, at this point in time dance therapy has achieved equal status with other health-related professions, and is now acknowledged as an effective form of treatment for individuals with a wide range of problems, from emotionally disturbed children and adults, through institutionalized psychiatric patients, to the subjects with whom we are dealing in this chapter: the elderly.

DANCE THERAPY GROUPS FOR THE ELDERLY

Every age group benefits from dance therapy. The elderly experience emotional and physical gains, proportionate, of course, to their declining physical abilities and impaired emotional health, and to the extent that they are living in institutional surroundings. The approach will depend upon the needs of the group. Through planned emphasis on self-awareness, communication, group interaction, and relaxation, dance therapy becomes a powerful therapeutic tool.

Dance for the elderly is now given a place in our culture as an important nonverbal means of communication and comfort. It is not surprising, therefore, that dance for the elderly is an established therapeutic modality. Dance therapy addresses the need for dance in the elderly, who are sometimes overcome by self-pity, inertia, and depression. Many elderly may feel the emptiness of not being needed anymore; of being near the end of their time on earth. Many have lost their sense of self-esteem, and these feelings are damaging to their mental and physical well-being. But when they dance, either holding hands or facing a partner, they regain a feeling of togetherness, of contact with others. Subconscious memories flood them: they are again vital and energetic. The rhythms take over their bodies and they forget their self-pity, body aches, ailments. Arthritic pains are eased by the movement. They feel young again. They feel worthy again. They do not feel they are "thrown-away" human beings. They feel they *belong!*

CHOICE AND BENEFIT OF ACTIVITIES

In commenting on the origins of dance, Franziska Boas noted (1971): "Each person has a basic rhythm of his own. . . . The movement itself may not be coordinated in the usual sense but a rhythmic coordination can be accomplished which gives pleasure to the dancer and the observer" (p. 23). This is especially applicable to therapeutic dance.

Dance movements need not be complete; they may be as simple as swinging arms, legs, or feet; stretching and reaching; rotating the head or upper torso from side to side; or even just clapping hands. Groups are varied, and the fitness of members depends not so much on chronological age as on the individual's abilities and disabilities; some may be regressed, others incapacitated. At the beginning, it is difficult to reach depressed or regressed group members. I use music or touch, or any of the sensory modalities. For the more energetic or more able, I use more energetic and vigorous activities.

The session may begin with a warm-up during which patients clap hands in time to music. I encourage the use of the whole body. Patients in wheelchairs, who cannot use their legs, are particularly encouraged to clap hands and effect some movement in their entire bodies. Use of the entire body involves the patient in more basic feelings.

An English authority on body image and ego development, Dr. Paul Schilder, correctly observed in 1925, "Movement is a great uniting factor between the different parts of one's own body" (p. 112).

Unquestionably, identifying the parts of the body through movement is useful for space disorientation and agnosia (an unawareness of body parts). One elderly gentleman with a partial stroke who could not move one side of his body and could say but one word— *Wunderbar*—became so animated that he would clap vigorously and sing loudly. By the way he said "Wunderbar" he revealed how excited and joyful he was at participating.

I have found that what may appear to be very simple actions have great potential for helping elderly patients who suffer from a variety of physical limitations related to the progressive deterioration of the aging body. Dance therapy is an especially practical and helpful form of treatment, because every patient, no matter how severely disabled, can participate.

For example, a man in his nineties who had had both of his legs amputated because of diabetes was able to take part in a dance session. Although at first he was unwilling to join in, he was encouraged to participate through whatever motions he could perform. Similarly, a blind woman in her late eighties was able to join in with the group because the therapist called out the motions so she could hear what the group was doing.

No matter what their disabilities, patients are able to participate at whatever level is comfortable. In so doing, they not only achieve the benefits of physical motion, but gain a sense that they are capable of doing things with ease and enjoyment.

It is important to realize that low-intensity movement has a great capacity for improving the elasticity of muscles and joints, and for relieving stress. Other forms of activity in dance therapy, such as individual or group dances, need not be vigorous, and are greatly enjoyed by the more able patients.

When I first came to the Jewish Home and Hospital for the Aged to work with patients, the doctors watched me intensely, fearful that the patients would overtax themselves and become exhausted or injured. However, by the end of the session everyone was so inspired and was having so much fun that the doctors had to agree that this was an excellent activity.

Built-up tension causes fatigue. Frustration, anger, and self-pity have a direct effect on muscles, ligaments, and the circulatory system. Sedentary positions cause muscles to contract, becoming painful and creating discomfort in all parts of the body. Because they tend to be sedentary and are susceptible to all types of anxieties, depression, and fear, the elderly may be helped by relaxation and breathing exercises. Such exercises, interspersed throughout the session, are barriers to fatigue and stress, and are always used at the end of the class for a quiet and relaxing cooling-off period. The two examples below are typical.

Mrs. A., an elderly woman at a nursing home, frequently informs me that whenever she has palpitations of the heart, she is able to slow down her heartbeat by doing the rhythmic breathing and relaxation exercises used in class.

Recently, a strike of hospital workers was about to be called. The residents of the various hospitals and old-age and nursing homes where I work were very agitated when I arrived. I tried to follow through with the session, but questions and fears were uppermost in their minds and concentration was poor. We spent most of the session discussing the various aspects of the impending strike and then followed through with the breathing and relaxation activity. The group relaxed then and was able to focus in on other activities.

PHYSICAL AND EMOTIONAL GOALS

Although physical goals are an essential part of dance therapy programs, equally necessary (though not most important) is the improved emotional health of the participants. It is vital to the elderly to offer them outlets for self-expression and opportunities for social interaction, physical activity, and relaxation.

The build-up of tension in the elderly also produces symptoms such as insomnia, fretfulness, and restlessness. Some of the elderly turn their resentments in upon themselves, and unrealized aggressive tendencies become self-directed and produce even greater stress, resulting in angry or depressed behavior.

We must remember that an elderly person often suffers the loss of independence, both financial and social; this in turn produces a loss of confidence, and then self-pity, passivity, frustration, and resentment. Sometimes the individual resorts to delusions or regressions in an effort to withdraw from an all too painful reality.

We must never lose sight of the fact that elderly persons are usually removed from their families; sadly, they may not be visited often enough, even by their children.

Many emotional disturbances in the elderly are caused by vascular and neurological diseases that cause personality changes, bringing about anxiety, withdrawal, confusion, depression, hyperactivity, irrational behavior, incontinence, forgetfulness, anger, and a constantly complaining and demanding style of interaction. Under these conditions, dance therapy group sessions for the afflicted elderly are an ideal means of discovering, preventing, arresting, and even reversing the damaging effects of aging. The movement therapist offers stimulation for constructive recall, reality contacts, and social interaction. Patients respond with improved memory, alertness, reality orientation, and judgment. Other benefits include stability, subdued anxiety, personal insight, acceptance, and improvement in self-esteem. As a social activity, dance therapy mobilizes patients who have become progressively immobile through the years. Dance group brings the elderly together in an accepting and encouraging atmosphere; it offers them a sense of belonging and, through contact with themselves and others, a sharpened sense of their own being. For instance, one woman, disgusted with her appearance, refused to join the group at first. But finally after she began coming to sessions, she brought out a record she had made years before, when she was a professional Yiddish singer. Many times, people who have never said much reveal their past in great detail after a few sessions.

THE IMPORTANCE OF DANCE THERAPY IN INSTITUTIONS

Marian Chace observed "patients in a hospital have exaggerations of the feelings of all people, but no difference in the feelings. Dance, then, is most valuable as a means of reducing the loneliness caused by these exaggerations of emotion and consequent increased separation from others" (1975, p. 203).

Dance therapy for the elderly is particularly important in residential facilities where the "sick role" seems paramount; these patients often withdraw from others, and they may engage in almost no significant interaction. A dance therapy group produces, even in the "sick" elderly, an improvement in social interaction. Interpersonal relationships are bettered because of the enormously pleasurable opportunity to increase adaptability, cooperation, and verbal and nonverbal communication. It is not uncommon for hostile or withdrawn patients, who may initially have resisted joining the group, to become more active members after only a few sessions. The following vignette illustrates this quite well.

Martha, who had been an accomplished painter, was already in the program when Sam entered it. Sam was very reluctant to stay, and I noticed during a session that he was very restless, several times to the point of almost leaving. But after a few sessions Martha took him under her wing, and he began to come in regularly. During the dancing part, he would come over to her, smiling, and begin to dance. His restlessness and "don't touch" attitude had altered radically. Now his smile and his active body revealed his enjoyment at being with Martha and the group.

Such positive results may extend to other activities and adaptive behaviors. Social workers report that after participation in dance therapy sessions their elderly clients were more likely to participate in arts and music programs, and responded better at meals and social events. The spillover that may be expected from dance therapy sessions is well illustrated in the following.

The residents of a nursing home seemed bored. A few were quarreling and screaming at one another when our session began. However, though I had expected the worst, the session turned out better than I had anticipated. The nurses and the attendants were stimulated to participate along with the residents. The singing, dancing, and talking continued long after the session was completed. It was all very exciting.

An important characteristic of the dance therapy experience is that even the smallest gains are in fact great accomplishments, much like getting a patient with a paralyzed leg to move just one toe even slightly. Often a resident may not appear to be participating. But when the session ends, she will tell me, much to my surprise, how much she has enjoyed the class. For example, a woman who sat almost comatose for several sessions eventually responded by waving her finger in time to the music. This was the first sign that she was aware of her surroundings, and after several more sessions she had progressed to the point where she would look up at fellow group members and shake hands.

Dance therapy is effective in overcoming one of the obvious symptoms of apathy and despair—immobility—as well as related symptoms such as nervous activity. Certain patients walk around in a frenzy, or constantly hit themselves or other objects. One goal in the sessions, therefore, may be to help patients direct their energy outward in positively channeled ways. One woman who was too restless to sit down through the warm-up movements began to participate in one of the dances, and from that time forward she attended regularly and was one of the most active members.

THE THERAPIST'S ROLE

The therapist's use of self with the group is vital to the success of the support session. The movement the therapist brings to the session is planned, but the therapist always remains flexible, as no two sessions are ever alike. By speaking with each member of the group individually, and touching an arm or shoulder where appropriate, the therapist helps group members feel wanted. Understanding and dedication are needed to look beyond the argumentative, sluggish, irrational, or unresponsive behavior of some patients, and to reach out to each individual's human qualities and needs.

Since elderly persons are sensitive to any hint of patronization or authoritarian behavior, it is necessary for the therapist to participate in the group as an active member, and to generate an atmosphere of giving, sharing, and accepting. Individual responses are welcomed without judgment or criticism, and each participant may refuse any activity. Gentle but firm encouragement is essential.

Touching

From cradle to grave, touching is a primary means of communication. When people approach old age, the need for it becomes intensified, for touching offers reassurance and helps ward off the "final separation"—the awesome realization that their time on earth must soon come to an end.

Adults discover the importance of skin contact in lovemaking, and when facing sexual problems tenderly massage each other before attempting the sex act. The elderly, especially those confined to institutions, hunger for human contact; sometimes the only avenue of communication is the sympathetic touch. The pity is that at this point in their lives, when the need is so great, they are not always as physically appealing as they were when younger. The elderly patient may get routine physical care but not enough gut-level human touch and warmth. Yet touching, or light massage, produces immediate positive responses. After just a little light touching, patients react immediately. One said, "I feel lighter, taller, and can even feel the wrinkles disappearing."

Often ambulatory patients are encouraged to touch patients who are less mobile. For the more depressed or regressed, it is sometimes far more reassuring and helpful to touch than merely to think.

Mirroring

Mirroring movements—which are reflective of emotions—are part of the dance therapy technique. This is seen in the case of a woman who cursed in Yiddish (which many staff members fortunately did not understand) and who would pinch me to let me know I could not turn my back on her. After several sessions in which I would mimic her actions, I was eventually able to get her to mimic me, and then alter her own movement and mirror a few of my motions. One of the valuable aspects of this technique is that without uttering a word a relationship is established with another individual.

Creativity in movement ideas is elicited and shared. For example, in a follow-the-leader dance or movement, one participant begins and then everyone gets into the swing of it. It is astonishing how much the participants can remember, and how much joy and satisfaction they derive from remembering and from doing.

Recently, after a successful session, an elderly man of about ninety-six came over to tell me that it wasn't so much what we did in the group as the interest I bring to it. He then told me that he had been a psychologist, and that he was now determined to continue to come to the sessions, as he enjoyed them so much.

One important difference between dance therapy for younger people and geriatric dance therapy is that in the former the therapy may be concerned more with long-range improvement; in geriatric dance therapy, by contrast, it is the joy of the moment that is important. And these moments may carry over into other activities and into relationships with others.

Mrs. B., who had been attending the sessions regularly, was invited to a radio show, along with a group of other elderly people, to discuss their feelings about aging. I was told later that they were sitting around the station when Mrs. B. suggested that as long as they were waiting why didn't they do Sonya's exercises. Sure enough, they all began to participate, as if they were in my class. The director of activities later told me how all the onlookers were impressed by the fact that not only did the elderly members remember the exercises, but that they helped them to relax.

With brain-damaged patients, too, the "joy of the moment" is meaningful. For instance, during a workshop on Alzheimer's disease at Gracie Square Hospital, I was demonstrating the use of dance movement when an elderly patient sitting with his family arose, walked over to me, put his arm around my waist, and proceeded to lead me in a dance. Soon his family and friends joined in with laughter as he danced smoothly and freely around the room.

CONCLUSION

Martha Graham once said that movement expresses emotions we cannot hide; in dance therapy, both positive and negative feelings should be permitted. Visitors to dance therapy sessions for the elderly are always amazed at the unexpected vitality, joy, and level of activity that characterizes most dance and movement sessions. In dance therapy groups, people have fun with one another. The therapy becomes a demonstration, even to the infirm, that their physical bodies need not be a burden to them but a source of pleasure, and that they may still experience the thrill of living.

REFERENCES

Boas, F. (1972), Origins of dance. In: *Dance Therapy: Roots and Extensions*. Columbia, Md.: American Dance Therapy Association.

Caplow-Lindner, E., Harpaz, L. & Samberg, S. (1979), *Therapeutic Dance Movement: Expressive Activities for Older Adults*. New York: Human Sciences Press.

Chace, M. (1975), *Marian Chace: Her Papers*, ed. Chaiklin. Columbia, Md.: American Dance Therapy Association.

Penfield, K. (1978), To dance is to learn to live again. *Therapy*. (Volume and page number unavailable).

Schilder, P. (1925), *The Image and Appearance of the Human Body*. England: Routledge & Kegan Paul.

19

Art Therapy Groups in a Geriatric Institutional Setting

JANE MORRIN, B.S.

Since its beginnings about forty years ago, art therapy has been concerned with the visual arts in the service of education, psychotherapy, and rehabilitation. This flexible modality can be offered individually or in groups to enhance the benefits and pleasures of creative expression. Because the psychotherapeutic interaction is partially nonverbal, an avenue of communication may be opened up, particularly for withdrawn patients.

It is generally accepted that the nonverbal expression of negative feelings in an artificial medium acceptable to others brings a release and relief of tension. Also, many procedures in art therapy are tailored to assist favorable changes in personality, based on the conviction that the forces involved in creativity are closely akin to those underlying the development of personality.

The art therapy experience can provide two different kinds of opportunity. One is for a single participant to express feelings safely within the confines of a structured nonverbal exercise with carefully limited goals, thereby enhancing the possibility of eventual verbal communication. The other occurs through the sharing of artistic creativity within a group; this may afford opportunities for more spontaneous patterns of interaction with the therapist, and with other members of the group, in what can become a therapeutic alliance.

As diagnostic tools, projective tests are now thoroughly accepted protocols. The Rorschach tests prepared the ground, and Murray's Thematic Apperception Test (TAT) has become an equally standard measurement. The Draw-a-Person and House-Tree-Person tests have also become familiar adjuncts in mental health practice. Similarly, the art therapist observes the participant's behavior and production in order to arrive at an understanding of the total personality, often in collaboration with a staff psychologist or psychiatrist. Since secondary elaboration can be a factor, as when a depressed patient uses only very bright colors, parallels can be looked for outside the activity (this is particularly true for the aged, who tend to use more pastel than primary colors).

On the other hand, as Kramer (1958) notes, the "habitually depressed or belligerent become amiable and cooperative while painting their monsters"; this affect of sublimation "shows that through painting [they] obtain temporary mastery over their conflicts so that the burden of anxiety and aggression is eased for them" (p. 87). In this situation, the art therapist pays close attention to the details of the patient's drawing for clues to problem areas. One picture being worth a thousand words, it can be useful for staff conferees to hear about the third eye or the sharp fangs of the monster.

It is the task of the art therapist to create conditions shaped to meet the needs of a specific individual or group. In many instances it may not be constructive to bring unconscious material too close to the surface through the suggestion of painful themes or the proffering of difficult insights. Such interference may trigger regression, which cannot always be handled usefully. An insightful art therapist who is also empathetic can convey without words the feeling that the unconscious meanings of the person's efforts are understood and accepted, but without bringing more of the material to consciousness than can be tolerated.

Recreation is an important need. In the preface to *Philosophy in a New Key* (1941), Susanne Langer quotes J. M. Thorburn: "All the genuine, deep delight of life is in showing people the mud-pies you have made; and life is at its best when we confidingly recommend our mud-pies to each other's sympathetic consideration" (pp. ix–x). Art therapy can provide great fun for groups in institutional settings, working within the capacities of the group.

Since art has much in common with dreams (Freud's royal road to the unconscious), and since painting provides an opportunity to project and socialize unconscious conflicts, sharing one's artwork with a group can be gratifying. The group will accept as a given that fantasy is not action, and the symbolic content of a work signals to the others some common emotional experience. If the group responds to the picture without censorship, a recognition of commonality is signaled. The artist's self-criticism is quieted as a result and he derives pleasure from the ventilation and discharge of tension while retaining self-control.

There is pleasure for the empathic viewer, too, in the sharing of the experience. It is in the viewing and limited discussion of the artwork that the support of the group is most valuable to both. And group support is invaluable for those who are basically isolated and afraid.

The art group in a geriatric setting offers group interaction to those whose lives have narrowed dramatically. It also provides latitude for independent decision making, a function necessarily curtailed in other areas.

An institutional resident should of course have the choice whether or not to participate. It is a given that patients are never pushed. Once having chosen to explore the art group, however, the joiner should find an atmosphere of playful warmth and encouragement, with emphasis on self-determination. The therapist must be equipped with some teaching skills in order to help the participant who wants to develop his artistic talents, but the quality of the product of creative expression should never be an important consideration. Aesthetics must give pride of place to the process of involvement and the building of self-confidence.

Art therapists in old-age and nursing institutions often work as members of interdisciplinary teams together with psychiatrists, psychologists, social workers, psychiatric nurses, and such others as physical therapists. Since art therapy involves some physical activity, it can help rehabilitate residents requiring muscle retraining or strengthening, or the improvement of coordination and range of motion.

A small group of six to eight people per session is best. Sessions should be from an hour to an hour and a half long. A suitable room with easy access to a water tap and wash basin, where supplies and works in progress can be stored safely, is important. One large table is best for accommodating wheelchairs and affords participants an opportunity to function as a group. Proximity encourages interaction.

Large sheets of paper may be intimidating; the 12" × 16" size is usually best. Crayons, oil pastels, pencils, and colored marking pens are good supplies with which to begin.

After greeting each member individually, the art therapist usually starts with simple assignments suggested because they require no ability or training in art. The penciled doodle, for example, is a good icebreaker: "Have you ever doodled while on the phone? Everyone's doodle is unique. Let's do some and see."

Precut cardboard shapes in assorted sizes can be distributed and traced to create a design to be colored. This works particularly well with patients with poor eyesight or motor impairment. String painting is another good exercise for the motor-impaired. Manageable lengths of cord are dipped into jars of tempera and then dragged across the paper. Bottle caps and other flat-bottomed objects dipped into the paint can be used to stamp colored shapes into the design.

Picture completion, a technique useful in work with disoriented patients, involves using whole figures cut from magazines and pasted down. Participants then color in an appropriate background, such as sky, sea, and sand behind a figure clad in a bathing suit. Drawing a simple household object—a cup, bowl, or flowerpot—after feeling its shape brings into play the sense of touch. This may be used to good effect with withdrawn individuals losing their grasp on reality.

A useful exercise encourages recall among those with impaired memory and helps maintain contact with a time of better-organized functioning. The titles used in the exercise are descriptive: "My Family Tree" (how many relatives do I remember?). "The Layout Where I Used to Live" (how were the rooms arranged?). "The Streets of My Old Neighborhood" (what were the names of cross streets?).

Of course there will always be those who resist structure, who insist on doing their own thing. This should be allowed. For the therapist, this stance and whatever is produced provide useful information which can be shared with staff.

As the above examples might suggest, art therapy is an extremely accommodating and flexible tool for therapy, both physical and mental. A perfect example which comes to mind is of a drawing done by a female member of a Golden Age Club in the Bronx. The exercise involved doing a loose scribble in pencil, then turning the paper around until some image was perceived among the lines and brought out by felt-tipped pen. The woman produced a drawing of herself as a young mother hugging her little girl, who as an adult was estranged from her. She cried, and the group, in trying to help her accept this sorrow, talked about their own difficulties in relating to offspring.

As this example shows discussion before the end of the session is vital to the art therapy process. But when time is up, residents should be encouraged to sign and date their drawings. Pictures hung up on the walls with care (and the painters' permission) can greatly improve self-esteem.

Space does not permit here a discussion of the places of the psychology of color and of symbol in art therapy. Suffice it to say that these are rich sources of information in diagnosis and prognosis. And for the participant, using color can be therapeutic. A reassuring comfort to the troubled, it is often a joy to us all.

A brief overview has been presented of art therapy rationales and techniques. But art therapy can include group mural painting, clay modeling, and other structural sculpting which may be equally rewarding.

Art therapy can be combined with other creative modalities, such as music therapy ("Listen to this music and then do a painting, realistic or abstract, as to how the music makes you feel"); movement therapy ("Let your arms move and your body sway to the beat of the music as you paint strokes in appropriate colors for the mood and rhythms of this piece"); and poetry therapy ("Do a picture, realistic or abstract, to communicate something of the poem which will now be read to you").

Current training in art therapy includes such disparate theoretical frameworks as Gestalt therapy, behavior modification, and client-centered and other humanistic therapies. But whatever the orientation, all art therapists have as their goals the provision of cathartic experience, the facilitation of impulse control, and the introduction of experiences designed to develop the ability to integrate and relate.

The following account of an art therapy session I led in an old-age home illustrates many of these points.

Mary, Sophie, Alvin, and Lillian had been in the group for months. Rachel was a comparative newcomer. The older members had decided on an ambitious project for the group just before Rachel joined them—a mural on a large sheet of oaktag which had been cut to fit comfortably on the table along with working tools and supplies.

They had decided to do a picture of a cheerful playground scene and had accumulated a store of photographs and illustrations of children. The best artists among them, Alvin and Lillian, who had been amateur painters even before becoming residents, were to copy these once the background was well under way. This strategy had been voted on, with the proviso that the others could try their hand at it as well.

A background of sky, trees, bushes, grass, and flowers constituted a kind of frieze across the top of the approximately 36″ × 28″ paper. This had been accomplished by painting verdant scenes on smaller sheets of paper, the best parts of which had been cut out and pasted across the top. It was quite effective.

Below the frieze, in pencil, the participants had sketched such things as swings, a seesaw, a sandbox, climbing bars, and climbing boxes in a stacked pile. At this session they planned to color in these various playground furnishings.

Mary, who had appointed herself my helper long before, arrived first and assisted me in setting out the supplies. She evidently enjoyed having me to herself and almost invariably arrived early, before the designated time of the session. I had found this comparatively vigorous seventy-year-old to be intelligent and insightful, but extremely sensitive to criticism from her peers. Years before, Mary had had two episodes of schizophrenia, from which she had recovered fairly well.

Gregarious Sophie and quiet Alvin arrived next. In her mid-seventies, Sophie was still a pretty woman who took care of her appearance with an obvious sense of style. She'd had a stroke which had affected her left side slightly some years before, but was clearly determined not to let it affect her social life.

By contrast, Alvin proclaimed by his behavior that he did not value socializing very much. Drawn to the group initially because it afforded him an opportunity to use the art supplies, this sixty-eight-year-old resident, who had had a series of heart attacks and suffered from emphysema, generally tried to be polite but would turn surly and pettish if pushed. His consenting to work on the mural had pleased me, as well as the other participants, very much.

Rachel came in next, and on her heels came Lillian in her motorized wheelchair. Rachel had joined the group upon the recommendation of her staff physician, who felt it would be beneficial for her both physically and emotionally. Suffering from a constellation of afflictions, including osteoporosis and palsy, Rachel was also somewhat antisocial. At this point, I felt that this seventy-eight-year-old might not stay long in the group, which so far had not accepted her.

The group was often impatient with Lillian, too, but her place in their midst was firmly established. Lillian was often difficult. In her midseventies, she had lost a foot to diabetes. Her eyesight had also been affected. This was frustrating for Lillian, who had been a gifted amateur painter. I assumed from her affect, however, that this intensely reactive person must always have been something of a whiner.

The verbal exchanges which follow are approximated from memory and shortened for brevity and emphasis. Also, some exchanges are lifted from previous sessions and included here for increased intelligibility to the reader.

Just as the group members got settled in their places after the usual bit of chatting, Rachel got up from her seat and hobbled with her cane to a window, muttering a little to herself as she looked out. The group chose to ignore her for the moment. I was going around the table, advising and assisting when asked, making sure without being mechanical about it that I said something personal to each member of the group.

"What a pretty scarf," I said to Sophie as I moved the bowl of water in front of her toward her good right side. (I made sure never to give a compliment I didn't mean.)

"Harry chose it for me. He had good taste," she replied in her slightly Russian-accented voice. Harry had been her third husband, whom she had married at seventy and lost at seventy-two. All three of Sophie's husbands had died during the course of her marriages.

Mary, next to her, agreed: "It's got beautiful colors."

Lillian, across the table, groaned immediately. Then, with everyone except Alvin looking at her, she said, "I don't feel so good. I should have stayed in bed this afternoon. I don't know why I'm here, anyway. I can't even see what I'm doing. I'm sorry I chose swings to do. I thought it would be easy on my eyes but I can't see what I'm doing, and anyway I'm not comfortable enough. It's too far away on the paper. I don't know what anybody expects from me!"

Alvin, with ruler and marking pen at his climbing bars (which appeared upside down from where he sat), said sotto voce to his hands, "Wonderful." His comment was ignored, except for Lillian's sucking at her dentures in anger. She'd learned from past clashes that getting into a fight with Alvin was a no-win proposition, so she was doing her equivalent of biting her tongue. (I privately considered this good coping strategy on Lillian's part, given the inevitable results of her irritability and its effect on others. She did have some impulse control, which was probably enhanced by her medication. I considered that it was this which explained her qualified acceptance by the group. What I was alert to were opportunities to afford her safe outlets to ventilate her rage, through abreaction, from historical causes of inner conflict. Such an opportunity arose later in this session.) In the meantime, I was busily rearranging the table to give Lillian better access to her drawing, and I connected a small desk lamp to an outlet in the wall to throw additional light directly on her area of work. I had previously found this to be helpful.

Next, with the members settled into their usual bantering around the table, I approached Rachel at the window. I was always careful never to touch her without her permission, although she often needed my hand to steady hers at the artwork. I stood quietly but not too close to her and asked if she was ready to get started.

"No."

"A little later then?"

"I can't do it."

"I'll help you."

"It's too hard."

"You'll see. It's not really difficult at all. We chose the sandbox because you agreed it was the easiest."

The sandbox had been drawn without perspective as a double rectangle, as if viewed from above.

Rachel gave me a wide berth as she hobbled past me toward the table. Although she wore a prescribed corset as support for her spine, it seemed to me she was more hunched over than ever. Her mutterings grew louder as she got closer to the table, and her head tremor increased.

"Silly. Just silly. What does he know? Supposed to be good for me? Ridiculous. Supposed to be a doctor? An idiot. Jerk. Dope. *Schle-miel*."

The table grew quiet momentarily. Alvin had finished his intricate black climbing bars and was sorting through the folder of photographs and illustrations of children. The plan was to paint them on separate pieces of paper and then to cut them out and paste them to the background.

Perhaps to fill the gap of silence, Mary said, "Oh, aren't they cute?" She had looked up from her climbing boxes, a stack of simple rectangles she was coloring in gay patterns, to what Alvin was doing. "I've been thinking of trying to copy a picture I have upstairs of my middle son, Joseph, in his confirmation suit. But I know I'd make a mess of it. For sure."

Sophie looked at what Mary was doing. "That's pretty," she commented. Then, looking down at the seesaw she was outlining with a brown marking pen, she made a deprecatory gesture at it. "That Joseph is your favorite son, isn't he?" she asked.

Mary stiffened. "Why do you say that? I love all three the same."

Sophie's eyes shifted. "Oh, I don't know. You talk about him the most."

"Do I? I didn't realize." She was flexing and rubbing her arthritic knuckles without, I believe, being aware of it.

"I think most mamas have a favorite child, maybe secretly, don't you?" Sophie asked tactfully. "My Selma, the younger one, is a real sweetheart."

"*I* agree," Lillian chimed in. "Now, Stanley has always been a good son. He writes to me every week faithfully from California, but Beth, living in Pennsylvania, well, that's another story. She's too much like me—running, running, always running." Then, realizing what she had said, Lillian laughed bitterly.

Rachel looked up at her. She was shakily dabbing a yellowish brown paint mixture in dots into her sandbox. I felt her look was empathic—a good sign.

"Years ago," Alvin volunteered uncharacteristically, "I thought maybe I made a mistake never getting married. But the more I hear, the more I'm glad I never had children." He was sketching a child in pencil on an 8″ × 10″ sheet of paper and using the ruler to measure it against the climbing bars. He was going to attempt pasting the sketch to the structure, I realized, pleased.

Mary was assisting Sophie's try at washing out a blotch of brown paint that had dripped from her brush accidentally, while they both spoke to Alvin about the pleasures of parenting.

Rachel interjected, "In a pig's eye!"

She was ignored.

"Well, how do *you* feel about children, Rachel?" I asked. My intervention was ignored and I considered that perhaps it was just as well. (*Careful, be careful,* I reminded myself.)

Lillian had completed her row of swings and reached up to turn off the lamp. "It comes back to me as if it was yesterday, Sam pushing Stanley in the swing when he was a baby and how Stanley loved it. Sam was a wonderful father, a good husband." Tears came to her eyes. "And now he's *gone.*" She sounded angry suddenly.

"You miss him a lot, don't you?" Mary asked. (Mary's ex-husband had remarried against his religion and she was bitter about that.)

Lillian was washing out her brushes. The group was starting to clean up now at my request. "I'm angry with him for leaving me," she admitted shamefacedly.

"He couldn't help it!" (Sophie, the veteran widow, sounded astonished.)

"What do you take me for, an idiot?" Lillian shot back.

"She knows that," Mary said quickly to Sophie. "But losing someone can feel like rejection, even if he passed away. You of all people ought to know that."

Sophie patted her coiffure thoughtfully. "So that's why I felt so peculiar when Sid was dying."

"It's a very common experience to feel conflicting emotions at such a time," I confirmed.

Alvin looked at me intently. "My mother . . . ," he started.

"Yes?" I said, thinking of the genesis of his distrust of women.

"I was just a kid," he said, breathing heavily.

"Yes, children especially feel deserted, abandoned, when a parent dies. It often makes them angry on top of the pain."

"So *that's* why Beth turned on me when her father had that heart attack," Lillian blurted out, twisting in her wheelchair. "She practically accused me of wearing him out, of causing it." Her face twisted as she searched for tissues in her pocket. "The nerve of her! She worried him plenty."

Mary, starting to cry as I moved to Lillian's side, said, "I found out in therapy that when my mother died, I felt guilty, too. She used to say that I was killing her."

Sophie got up and put her arms around Mary. I was comforting Lillian with half an eye on Rachel, who stared into her lap.

As if it were being dragged out of her, Lillian said, "Maybe I did feel a little guilty for Sam's heart attack." She was crying bitterly. "I *was* always wanting us to go, go, go."

Rachel got up and, leaving her materials as they lay, hobbled toward the exit. Failing to catch her eye, I said to her, " 'Bye, now. See you next week, Rachel."

"Good-bye," she responded civilly, without looking at me as she went out the door. I felt reassured by that, however, and by the thoughtful but not distracted look on her face.

Lillian and Mary had stopped crying and now Lillian laughed relievedly. "It's crazy, but I feel better now, like a load is off my chest. Somehow I feel less afraid of dying myself now."

Mary smiled and said, "Me, too."

Alvin leaned over and patted one tap to Mary's shoulder, a "good for you" kind of tap.

Depending on the level of functioning within the ongoing group and upon the skills of the group leader, it is not always advisable to have a discussion in depth at the end of a session, though it is an important part of therapy to have the attention and concern of the whole group focused on each member in turn, and members' critical faculties will be stimulated by their having to formulate and articulate their reactions. The training and ability of the therapist in assessing the effect of such discussion on individuals comes into play here.

Nevertheless, since reminiscence and life review are common preoccupations among the elderly, it is very helpful to them to be afforded opportunities to talk about loss, grief, decline, and death. In art therapy as in general, modifications of the psychotherapeutic approach make good sense when working with the aged. Environmental manipulation may be necessary and the art therapist must be more physically active and less psychically ambitious, using educational techniques to assist enhancement of self-esteem whenever possible. Resistance and transference must always be handled delicately, and respect for the accumulated affect of each adult participant's lifetime maintained. Respect cannot be faked, and cues can be picked up from the wisdom of the group as a unit. There is much to be learned from it.

A final aim of art therapy is to help patients develop and enjoy art skills at their own pace as an outlet for emotions. Although *art* may be conceded to be the province of artists, the kind of imagination essential to art may be widely distributed, coming to expression in *art* only under special conditions of motive and opportunity. Characteristics of the creative imagination have appeared throughout history in the design and ornamentation of objects in practical use.

Creativity is not a function of intelligence as measured by I.Q. tests. For certain creative activities, a minimum I.Q. is necessary, but beyond that artistic sensibility can be encouraged to find visual expression for feelings, without the good and bad connotations of words, which sometimes obscure true meaning for speaker and listener alike.

REFERENCES

Kramer, E. (1958), *Art Therapy in a Children's Community: A Study of the Function of Art Therapy in the Treatment Program of Wiltwyck School for Boys*. Springfield, IL: Thomas.

Langer, S. K. (1941), *Philosophy in a New Key: A Study in the Symbolism of Reason, Rite, and Art*. Cambridge: Harvard University Press.

Thorburn, John M. (1925), *Art and the Unconscious*. London: Kegan Paul, Trench, & Trubner.

20

Drama Gerontology: Group Therapy Through Counseling and Drama Techniques

RONICA STERN, Ed.M., M.A.

"Acting is doing something real in an imaginary circumstance." Through my two decades of professional experience in the theater and working intergenerationally with students eager to gain insights and heightened awareness of characterization in the many roles an actor is expected to explore, this statement stands as a canon.

It is second nature for the actor to be aware of the importance of ensemble acting. Whether the Group Theater of the thirties, Stanislavski's Moscow Art Theater, or the Old Vic, repertory demanded interaction and interpersonal relationship. The "as if" of acting was predicated on understanding and caring for one another. The focus of performance wed the ensemble company to fusion.

This immersion is achieved in a subtle weaving of interior and exterior exploration. It includes sensory work and detailed exposition of feelings. And it is permissible, because it is seen as "fleshing out" the character in the scene and not as a violation of the vulnerable self. It is the road to resolution.

These introductory remarks are mandatory if the reader is to be made aware of how easily theater techniques can transfer to the socialization and increased mental agility of the elderly. Since 1976 I have worked with older adults in a variety of circumstances. Whatever the title given these courses and workshops, my hidden agenda has always been to motivate groups and facilitate their cohesion so that members can function as support systems for one another. If loss is the inevitable gift of time, why not face it together, helping each other along the way? Theater techniques facilitate the journey. The importance of specificity of focus, motivation, purpose, obstacle, and resolution are all marshaled toward a common goal. "The play's the thing!" And, indeed, in theater production all forces unite, technicians as well as the visibly creative actors, to mount the piece.

The same case can be made for the "drama of life." If staff (technicians) and older adults (the actors) create supportive environments for the exploration of purposeful endeavor, a lifelong process of growth and learning is attainable. How we vary our actions, allowing ourselves to be leading players in our lives, is what is "acted" upon in the group workshop.

In the following pages I will give specific examples of work done with four groups of elderly persons. Though the basic techniques remain essentially the same, circumstances and the population change the value of the work dramatically in terms of how it is administered and how it is received. It changes, as well, if it is not supported by staff and coordinated with other institutional programs. Progress depends on consistency in attendance and concentration on the here and now. Momentum is lost if the workshop is scheduled at the same time as an outing is planned or if the podiatrist, dentist, etc. elects to come to see patients at the exact hour of the workshop. Older adults have lived with the medical model as prime consideration far longer than with concerns for quality of mind.

These caveats, of course, pertain to the institutionalized elderly. Elderly in the community, who avail themselves of courses given at senior centers or local libraries, also fall heir to erratic bus scheduling, smorgasbord samplers of courses rather than ongoing development, and so on. I cannot state the case too strongly. If *quality of mind* is a goal to be realized for our aging population, then courses which stimulate the thinking process should be treated as respectfully as other, mandatory therapies.

In January 1978 I gave a course entitled "Choices for Change" at the Jewish Institute of Geriatric Care in New York. It was funded for nine weeks and was repeated for another nine weeks because of the positive response. Then the grant ran out and the workshop was over. Although I had worked with older adults in the community using drama, this was my first experience in an institutional setting. I was given a clear space in an open lounge. Patients lined the walls, eyes glued to the television. It appeared to be a kind of mass hypnosis that Svengali might have found useful. The activities director and an aide helped me move people into a circle. I waived the use of a microphone. It discourages intimacy and connectedness.

"But what happens if someone is hard of hearing?"

"We'll have to listen harder."

That may sound flip or callous, but I have seen concentration and attention serve the hard of hearing better than the booming mechanism that separates one from the group and intimidates would-be participants.

I introduce myself and explain that we will use drama exercises to get to know each other better. We are a group of people meeting for the first time in a special way. Do they know each other's names? Not many do, they admit. So how are we to remember? A name, I tell them, is merely a toy. Most times, not even of our own choosing. A handy reference for a complicated chemistry. But inside that name is an essence. A quality which is memorable. Is the woman gracious, aggressive, shy, or calculating? Is the man overbearing, retiring, eager, or tyrannical? If we respond to the quality, allow it to affect us, the name of the person may not always come to mind but the person's essence is with us always. It is now in our emotional memory. Much as the berry-stained favorite dress worn to a picnic you have not thought of in years. Not until you taste a blueberry which falls from your lips spreading just such a stain evoking the earlier hidden memory.

The exercise extends itself. Each participant bestows a quality on the person opposite. The person can accept the quality or decide he/she is something quite different. Spin-offs can prompt questions and further exercises:

How many persons are you?

Are you one kind of person at one time, one place, or to one person, and different other times, places, or to different people?

How does it feel to be perceived as someone powerful when you feel you are powerless? Talkative when you feel you are reticent?

What name would you have liked to have?

In an opening statement say something to your partner with the quality your partner says you have.

And we are on our way to improvisation with emphasis on a simple purpose, the obstacle that prevents resolution and the choices we have that may overcome that difficulty.

In subsequent weeks I can remember problems worked on improvisationally that included the roommate who wanted the window open though her partner wanted it kept closed. A woman who wanted to go home though there was no one to care for her there. And wonderful Kata, who was deaf and sat at my side and wrote out a sense memory of her garden in Germany which she read to everyone after many sessions. Prior to the group's convening, she had remained in her room convinced she could contribute nothing.

When the program ran out of funds I visited Kata on my own. She had taken to writing many of her memories down and was eager to share them. Have I mentioned she was ninety years of age and had never married? She had been a housekeeper most of her life, taking care of other people's families.

I came back to the fifth floor and was greeted warmly by former members of the group. No similar program had replaced the work. A volunteer sat in the center of the lounge singing old-time songs. She encouraged the patients to join in. Few did. Most of the people were in their wheelchairs lined up against the wall, the familiar battlement, their staring, vacant eyes once more fixed on the television, volume lowered in deference to the "entertainment."

One of the senior centers I worked in was in a working-class neighborhood in Queens. There was the usual "all-purpose" room. I can understand the financial and even the social benefits of such an arrangement. But though budgetary rewards accrue for building one open space rather than rooms which allow for concentration and study, socialization is not the automatic response. This neighborhood reflected changing ethnic demographics dramatically. The retired postal worker, fireman, German, Irish, and Italian housewives stayed at their respective oblong tables working handicrafts or playing cards. Jamaican blacks sat separately doing beading and indigenous crafts. One of the first things I did was to push back the oblong tables and have everyone join a circle. Not everyone joined at first, but seventeen did. I still have the list. It was the first time, the director said, that the members were sitting side by side, black and white. The icebreaker we used was an immediate success. People of all ages like to play games.

"We are an acting company," I explained. "We are going on a tour, a national road company, and in our trunk (a magic trunk) we took—" Rules of the game follow. The actor must say his name loud and clear and place in the trunk an object (tangible, intangible, philosophic, etc.) that bears the first letter of the actor's first name. Having stated name and object, the second person adds on the name and object of the person before him, and so on. "It helps your memory, makes you a listening partner and shows off your imagination. Everything that's needed to be a fantastic showman and an interesting person!" And we're off.

The list tells me that Frank put in the F train; Catherine put in cats; Helen, a ham sandwich; Edith, eggs (in case we get hungry on the train—everyone laughed); Viola, a violin; Michael, money (everyone agreed—mighty necessary); Leoline, lilies; Hazel, a hat; Sybil, samples; Eva, energy (everyone thought this a wonderful choice); Phillipa, a piano; August, an anvil; Mabel, magic tricks; Isabel, Ivory soap—and you get the idea. If the person ran through the repetition without error there was wild applause and the flush of victory. If there was faltering, everyone cheerfully supplied the missing object or name. After sixteen repetitions "I couldn't do that" became "that was fun—I didn't know I could do it!"

In succeeding weeks the group got to know more and more about each other. An exercise called "What do you know?" brought forth these responses:

Catherine: I know laughter.

Anne: I know how to love people.

Edith: I know I feel good today. No pain.

Leoline: When people call and I'm still in bed, I clear my throat and make believe I've been up for hours.

The group smiles warmly in recognition. We tell each other fact as well as foible. We listen and use much of what we hear and know in the improvisations we work on at the end of each session.

This course too is extended for a second nine-week stint, and then "out with the garbage." No more grant money. The members are unhappy. They'll miss the fun, the learning, the stimulation. The director is equally desolate. "But what can we do? The first money is always needed for hot lunches and transportation. After that, we rely on volunteers." Unhappily, I too require lunches (hot or cold). Off goes "Ronica Drama-seed."

I have promised to highlight only four of the programs but before going further, reference has to be made to courses given in the past where, commendably, time slots were proportionately justified for constructive measures of growth and contributed incalculably to the goals inherent in the tenets of this form of drama therapy.

The goals set before the group and agreed to by consensus were:

To maintain an atmosphere in which common concerns could be freely discussed and in which members could interact with one another.

To provide and encourage the opportunity to voice complaints and to include members in decision making processes affecting the group focus.

To listen to one another. ("Listening is the beginning of understanding; everybody counts.")

To proceed in one's *own* way, understanding that in improvisatory work there is no right way and no wrong way (ideas hard to erode).

To accept that criticism is valid when it is not labeling but descriptive of behavior.

To develop flexibility and to promote risk taking.

To encourage sharing of experiences through speaking and listening, acting and reacting.

To support emotional investment in other people. ("If you give you'll get.")

To debunk myths regarding the elderly.

To remind ourselves that feelings are facts to the person "feeling."

In sites where the course structure ran from sixteen weeks to more than two years, the group performed original material, Feiffer's People, sketches from The Thurber Carnival, and scripts culled from experiences within the center they attended.

In other situations, where the obligation to perform was not "product-oriented," the group continued to explore in terms of contemporary issues and global concerns—just about anything anyone wished to discuss. Out of the ease of group support and an atmosphere of encouragement, discussion was free flowing. Argument, an opposite point of view, was immediately the premise for an improvisation with the contending roles reversed. This may not always have resolved the argument, but it went a long way in terms of "walk a mile in my shoes."

In 1982 I was hired as a drama workshop leader for a large senior center in Brooklyn serving over six hundred people daily. Thirty-five people signed up for the workshop. Not more than two or three knew each other's names or had more than a nodding acquaintance with one another. Yes, they had taken some courses together, but "you go, you listen to the teacher, and that's it—you don't really *talk* to anyone."

At the time, I was in a Teachers College master's program in counseling psychology, with a concentration in gerontology. How many students did I talk to in classes? In this center, we were given a room which was divided from other space by an accordion divider. The room was stuffy—no windows, no air conditioning. It had a huge fan that created so much noise few of the participants could be heard above it. We kept the doors open. Intimacy and connectedness was won by telling passers-by that no, they could not just come in and watch. Later there would be additional registration. For now, the group was confined to the people who originally signed up.

This was an unusually large group, and in subsequent sessions the number never went under twenty-eight in attendance. I held two-hour sessions and was determined that everyone would have a chance to work.

We added to our original set of rules. Here, the director of the center wanted a production of some kind. The social worker was a little more progressive. She assured me she understood work in terms of improvisation and that the end product need not be a formal one. Original sketches out of experiential happenings would be fine. But would it? If, in the work I hoped to do, I could get people to interact with insight and awareness, to trust each other, touch each other, be honest with each other, would they willingly disclose sensitive, reve-latory portraits of their persona for "production" purposes?

In the first and second sessions much attention was focused on *process*. How our group would operate. This required the delineation of guidelines and statements repeated many, many times. I had Xe-roxes made so the material could be studied, but I knew we had to have explanation and discussion. In addition to the goals listed above, we added:

To generate supportive behaviors.

To listen empathically.

To be honest.

To be open to new experiences.

To be open to how one is perceived by others.

To be imaginative. To go as far as one cares to in fantasy.

To be as real as one has to be in concrete situations.

To remember, above all, that acting is doing something *real* in an imaginary situation.

To relate to an object, a place, or a partner with real feelings about that object, place, or partner.

To *care*, in life as well as on the stage.

To have fun.

In order to impart group feelings of sharing I used nonsense songs. "Poisoning Pigeons in the Park" by Tom Lehrer was an ex-cellent choice. They learned to start and finish together; to listen to each other so they could come in at the right time; to say nonsensical things and not feel self-conscious; to have a good time while aiding articulation, projection, and coexistence in a large workshop; to fulfill the dictum "everybody counts."

We worked on improvisations that underscored many theoretical concepts of interpersonal growth. Rogerian theory speaks of congruence: facial expression and body language must match the verbal message or else the receiver gets mixed signals. Empathy and reflective support can be constructive tools in communication. There is a wealth of experience that can be shared and empathic listening can overcome factors that create schisms. We don't have to be equal; we merely have to respect the fact that each of us is different and that that is all right.

As actors and as members of the group we had the responsibility to be sensitive to conditions of mood and place. Did we feel the same at different times of the day (dawn, noon, sunset)? Interior and exterior conditions change a message. A headache (interior condition) or a bewildering atmosphere (exterior condition) changes the tenor of a conversation. And—a final cautionary note—in improvisation, as in life, the message should be relevant, explicit, honest, and not monopolized by a single participant.

Many incredible and wonderful things happened during the eight months we worked together. It is impossible to include all of them, but a few will perhaps suffice.

In the ninth session after a sensory exercise rubbing backs against each other, Jeanette said, "I felt I was being rocked gently in the uterus." To this Matthew, reserved and very proper, replied: "In the beginning I wasn't relaxed in the touching exercises; after all, we were men and women. Then we got to be friends and it was okay."

In the exercise "What was the hardest thing to give up?" the following interchange took place:

Ruth: (straightforward) An antique from my mother. My two sisters wanted it, but I wouldn't give it up.

Max: My "immaturity."

The final group was a mixture of sighted and blind frail elderly which met at a nursing home, funded through a grant given by La Guardia Community College. Here the emphasis was shared learning by blind and sighted elderly, the two populations who do not often socialize. The course of study was ambitious. We reviewed excerpts of plays by Sophocles, Chekhov, Ibsen, O'Neill, Williams, and Miller. But always, the emphasis was to provide the opportunity for interaction. We used improvisation, discussion, analogy, and personal experiences to analyze themes. Pride and destiny's hapless twists in *Oedipus* had immediate resonance in the group. There was immense pleasure in remembering plays. Memories ignited, and there would be recollections of great character actors and evenings in the theater. Learning about the authors and the society in which they lived and wrote was exciting. But many of the participants wanted to perform as well. And in the next eight weeks these frail elderly participants put on an admirable production of a short story by Isaac Bashevis Singer. The enthused activities director helped with costumes and beards for our chorus of elders. *Everyone* participated, some with lines and some with broad and humorous gestures. We put the show on twice, once for the skilled nursing facility and once for the health-related facility next door. The participants and the audience had a wonderful time. Here too there was pride in being part of a shared dramatic experience of intellectual significance.

An observer of the workshop had this to say: "These class members tend to have a poor self-image as handicapped individuals. Participating in an educational experience such as this one shows them their intellectual capacities, raises their own expectations for themselves, and enhances their self-image."

This program too was funded for two nine-week sessions only. Because work of this kind is not mandated at senior care facilities, as is physical and occupational therapy, outside funds on limited grants do not allow for the long-term progression required to nurture trust and affiliative growth patterns.

It is to be profoundly wished that mental stimulus and programs of participation that encourage positive relationships and peer support systems will become as important and necessary as we deem "concrete services." Lifelong educational pursuits enhance the quality of life. We are living longer. We should be given the skills to allow us to enjoy the increment.

Part VI
Training

21

Using Group Training Methods to Prepare
Students for Group Work with Older Adults

CONSTANCE MOERMAN, M.A.

The Adult Health and Development Program (AHDP): Working with Senior Citizens. Mental Health 212X, an exploratory interdisciplinary course. Provides training and experience in a personal growth-oriented program for older adults. Emphasis is on learning therapeutic skills and attitudes, theoretical knowledge, and practical applications for working with these clients on a one-to-one basis and in small groups. Consists of a three-hour per week seminar on the psychosocial and physical aspects of aging in America, a four-hour per week laboratory experience working with clients who will be drawn from the surrounding communities, and a 75-hour field placement at a senior day care center or nursing home.

This is the catalog description of a specialized training course which is part of the two-year Mental Health Associate (M.H.A.) curriculum at Montgomery Community College in Maryland. Started as an exploratory course in 1979, it has become an important part of training for students who want to work in the growing field of gerontology.

Growing old in America is becoming the "in" thing to do. The population explosion is in the upper age levels—in the 1980 census,

I wish to acknowledge Dan Leviton, Ph.D., of the University of Maryland, whose original creation of the Saturday morning Activity Program for Older Adults at the University of Maryland, run by graduate students, served as an inspiration for developing the training program at Montgomery Community College (see Leviton, 1975).

11 percent of the population was over sixty-five. Characteristically, the American way is to "do something" about every emerging problem. Legislation has been passed and a criss-crossing mesh of services for the elderly has been provided. The emphasis has been on doing "for" and "to" the elderly, largely because aging has been defined almost entirely in terms of the sick and the needy. However, 95 percent of the elderly (those sixty-five or older) live in their own homes, leaving only 5 percent to be cared for in institutions. Thus, most of the elderly can be quite actively engaged in society.

In creating the Adult Health and Development Program, I wanted to emphasize the growth potential of getting older, to demonstrate that the quality of life could improve—it does not have to go downhill if one takes charge of it. The overall goal of the program is to improve or maintain the physical health and emotional well-being of the older adult members in the program, and to help students develop the skills, attitudes, knowledge, and sensitivity necessary for working therapeutically with this population.

We had two main tasks to accomplish before we could work with our clients: (1) to begin training the students; and (2) to find our clientele, who would be known as Club Members of the Montgomery Community College Adult Health and Development Program. We allotted ourselves a month to train students in basic skills and to interest older citizens in our program. The class, consisting of twenty-one students, two instructors, and the director of the M.H.A. program, was scheduled to meet four hours per week in our physical education facility and three hours per week for the seminar on aging in a regular classroom. The students in this initial group were at various levels in their M.H.A. training. Some had taken the introductory group dynamics and mental health skills classes, while some were entry-level students with nine to thirty general education credits. Their age range was eighteen to sixty. There were males and females and representatives from three different races and several ethnic groups. Since our clients would also be coming from various cultures and ethnic backgrounds, we considered the heterogeneous student group a plus that promised a variety of skills and experiences.

We used two texts which suited our humanistic philosophy and also contained the necessary theory and information, presented at a suitable educational level for community college students. Many texts emphasize facts and figures rather than people. The two we selected, described below, were ideal for our purposes:

The first, *A Time to Enjoy: The Pleasures of Aging* by Dangott and Kalish (1979), emphasizes the positive, growth-related aspects of aging without ignoring the difficulties. It includes biological facts, statistics, and developmental tasks we face as we grow old. It addresses how to prevent physical deterioration by selecting healthy habits and how to promote emotional well-being. The focus is on aging as a time for new experiences and changing attitudes about self-image.

The second was *Working With the Elderly: Group Processes and Techniques* by Burnside. Burnside uses her rich experience in social-psychiatric services for the elderly to demonstrate the use of groups in improving their quality of life. It is essentially a how-to book, heavily weighted toward the operational aspects of group work rather than toward theories of group dynamics. However, there is sufficient material about the theoretical frame of reference and the history of group work with the elderly for the objectives of our program.

A brief description of how we incorporated the theoretical and biological aspects of the course with group learning experiences and practical applications to real live clients follows.

THE TRAINING PROCEDURE

The first month of training, before our clients arrived, was divided into two sections focusing on different aspects of the training program: Applied-Experiential and Didactic-Theoretical.

Section I was essentially a learning-by-doing-and-being practicum, meeting in the physical education facility. Its main purpose was to prepare students for hands-on group work with their clients. The weekly sessions started with an hour and a half of group dynamics experience, preceded by a brief physical warm-up to music. The T-group was experiential, with no discussion of theoretical questions. The goals were to develop trust, cohesiveness, communication skills, and subgroup team building. This session was followed immediately by a brief discussion of what had taken place in group, including explanation of the dynamics and how they would apply to our elderly clients-to-be.

After a brief break, we continued with an hour-long lecture-discussion of the physical aspects of aging—both strengths and limitations. The remaining time, usually about an hour, was devoted to instructing students in the use of the equipment in the physical education facility. This was in response to anxieties expressed about using equipment incorrectly or with the wrong client.

Section II, also meeting once a week, functioned on a seminar model. Current information and theories about aging were discussed, as well as values and attitudes regarding it. A considerable amount of time was spent on learning by experience how to form small task groups to prepare activity sessions for clients.

Meanwhile, students and faculty were also busily combing the community for club members. And we found them—in senior residences, through church organizations, newspapers, radio interviews, friends, older relatives, nursing homes, and county agencies, and through our announcements, which papered the community.

PHILOSOPHY AND FRAME OF REFERENCE

There are strong feelings among higher level professionals, who are zealously guarding their turf, about who should be doing group work with the elderly. Some caution that nonprofessionals may release strong feelings in the group that they won't be able to handle. But as Burnside writes in the preface of our text,

> We sell the elderly short; they are a tough lot. The danger is not in the practice of group work with the elderly. The real danger is in *not* conducting groups and thereby fostering the still prevalent "therapeutic nihilism" attitudes. It is better to take a risk than to sit by and watch the apathy, fear, sensory deprivation, loneliness, and helplessness continue in the aged. [p. xiv]

She speaks from a wealth of experience with this population and a knowledge of the great dearth of trained group workers in the field. We therefore limited our training objectives to imparting interventions, skills, and attitudes that would be effective in work with this population but could be learned in one semester.

The early emphasis in the program is on experiential learning —learning about group practice by being a group. Our model and frame of reference is fundamentally an interpersonal orientation based on Schutz's interpersonal needs theory (1960), reenforced with some of Yalom's theories about the curative factors of groups (1975). Those most relevant to group practice with the elderly are cohesion, universality, interpersonal learning, catharsis, identification, and hope.

Cohesiveness and universality are especially important for the elderly, who are constantly losing friends and relatives. To learn that their peers are having the same experience and can share their feelings is very reassuring. Catharsis is especially important for residents in institutions. The group becomes a safe place where they can vent their feelings about management, and the group meeting inspires hope as it becomes something to look forward to and count on each week.

Schutz's theory is based on the notion that most people have three basic interpersonal needs or desires—inclusion, control, and affection—which they both express toward others and want reciprocated. In training our students, we stress the significance of these needs by making them aware of their own needs in the training group. However, in working with the elderly, interventions are stressed differently from those in psychodynamic group psychotherapy.

Inclusion. For example, it is most important to include each member in each group meeting. The leader should not "wait out" the silent member. Eye contact, greetings, physical closeness, drawing the silent ones into the discussion, "going around," a friendly pat or hug, are all important.

Control. This is a delicate balancing act. Older people in institutions keep losing more and more control over their lives, usually after many years of making all of their own decisions. The group can become a place of empowerment where decisions can be made about their participation and relationships in the group. New group leaders can become very discouraged by the passivity, depressions, and dependence of many of these clients. Our students are told to expect this, so we try to stimulate them to be quite active in their groups and to develop ways of involving their clients in the group process. Sometimes they may have to complete group tasks so that the members can have a sense of accomplishment, even if they were unable to complete the task themselves.

Affection. Affectional and intimacy needs are an important component of group work with the elderly. In our training program we bring these needs into awareness by establishing an intimate affectionate environment in the student training group. Part of the method is for each student, when the clients join the program, to be assigned to one or two individuals in whom he or she will take special interest—telephoning them during the week, observing birthdays, being responsible for their activities at the college.

And so we readied ourselves for the arrival of our clients. Finally, after a month of intensive training for the students, they arrived.

Membership grew steadily until we had twenty-four members. Then word got around that something special for senior citizens was happening on our campus, and we now have a waiting list.

The students were eager to learn techniques. But it wasn't until they had experienced actual interaction with the members that they realized that *what* they did was not nearly so important as *how* they did it—that almost any technique administered with love and honesty and genuine attention to the client would work.

The first meeting, a plenary session, brought together in the gymnasium twenty-one students, twenty-four seniors, and three faculty. I introduced myself briefly, welcomed the seniors to the campus, and then, without further talk, initiated some group-building exercises. We formed a huge circle and did some easy stretching and breathing exercises. Everyone had been instructed to wear sneakers and comfortable clothing. We finished the session doing a very simple Greek dance to familiar music from *Zorba*. People were instructed to find someone in the group whom they did not know but who appealed to them for any reason. Seniors were instructed to find a student and students a senior, with faculty members filling in with the extra clientele. The members of each dyad were then to interview each other for about five minutes about interests, living space, retirement, educational plans, family, and why they had decided to participate in this experience, after which they were to return to the larger group and introduce their partners to the group. This was a free-for-all in which group members were encouraged to comment briefly or to ask questions of each other about what they had heard. There was a general sharing, after which we broke up into four smaller groups of six dyads each. The groups were randomly formed with only one restriction: no more than one faculty member to a group. After forty-five minutes we came back together, and each small group reported to the larger group how they had used the time to get to know one another and what they had observed about group process. The faculty members facilitated this process.

Then we announced the program for the rest of the morning. Three activities were offered: swimming for those seniors who had brought medical releases; yoga; or an exploratory walk around the campus and its environs. Students stayed with their seniors and participated with them in an activity. The seniors left at about twelve-fifteen, after which faculty and students assembled for forty-five minutes of feedback, summing up, and critical discussion. The processing periods immediately after a morning's activities were a very important training ingredient, as they gave students and faculty a specific time to explore what had gone on while the experience was still fresh. These sessions were intended to be participatory for all members, and as the semester went on and the students became clearer about their own goals and objectives, as well as those of the program, they became a most important aspect of the training.

For the next ten weeks seniors and students got together on Wednesday mornings from 9:15 to 12:15. The students continued to attend the three-hour Monday morning seminar. Within this time frame our program remained quite flexible as we learned more about what talents and skills our students and seniors had, what kinds of activities worked, and which ones were preferred. However, we didn't want to be so busy and so structured that there was no time for simple unplanned human relations. The Wednesday plenary session—students, seniors, and usually one faculty member—started with a half-hour warm-up led by two students using recorded music. (Later we discovered some musical talent in the group and frequently had live music for our activities.) Then the group broke up into small groups for three-quarters of an hour. These small groups were led by two students, who had usually prepared a focus for the meeting. Topics were frequently suggested by the seniors, some of whom had special expertise. Grandparenting, feelings about retirement and other life changes, the sharing of family pictures, planning an activity for the small group, making a group collage, current events, reminiscing, or just being together without a plan were topics and activities to which the small groups devoted themselves. I would always stay through this first hour and a half so that I could help give some cohesiveness to the community and help supervise the small group meetings. The other faculty member, whose special training was in therapeutic recreation for the elderly, would share time between two groups to give support to the students, as did I, but we did not intervene except as group members.

The remaining two hours were divided into two activity periods led by the students. Seniors would select from such offerings as water activities, yoga, modified aerobics, folk dancing, crafts, walks, movies relevant to the seniors' interests, and so on. There was never enough time for all of the possibilities, but we learned which activities were most appreciated and which led to personal growth and awareness.

In the Monday morning seminar we began to spend less time on didactics and theoretical discussions and more on planning for the Wednesday sessions with the clients through small group meetings, practice presentations to the whole class, troubleshooting, and some pretty heated meetings with feedback about performance. As in all groups, there were those who did their share or more and those who didn't. We tried to handle these issues within the Monday seminar. This did not always work and sometimes it was necessary to counsel one of the task groups or to meet with some of the students during my office hours for individual counseling.

WHAT HAPPENED TO THE STUDENTS

Within a few weeks, the students were able to take more and more responsibility for the Wednesday sessions. They were surprised by their own capabilities and ability to grow. All had a chance to test their leadership and followership skills, since those who weren't taking charge of an activity were participating in it along with their clients. They became more open in their relationships with each other and with their clients. Many reported that as they became more self-aware and self-confident their attitudes toward "the elderly" also changed. Following are some comments from a few of the students' course evaluation sheets:

"I've always had all of these negative feelings about older people. I felt it was time to learn who and what they really were. I wanted to get rid of my prejudices."

"I accomplished actual confrontation with older people in a day-care type setting. It was better than just book learning. I'm not afraid to face a group now or to try out new things with them."

"I liked the interaction between all of us. I liked the way we did not treat the older people as patients, but as members of our group."

However, working in the nursing homes to which they were assigned was more challenging than working in the "safer" atmosphere of the college gymnasium with a different kind of client. Our Senior Club members were living independently in the community, either alone or with a spouse or friend. They had made the effort to improve their daily experience by signing on to an experimental program. Most of them had gotten to the school on their own steam. The atmosphere was open, lively, and flexible, in contrast to the highly structured, coldly authoritarian ambience of many nursing homes. Frequently, institutional apathy and rigid programming had to be confronted. But our students did have many successes and were highly appreciated in these facilities. Every semester activity directors of the institutions call my office for student interns and to offer jobs to graduates. Burned-out nursing staffs and hard-pressed activity directors learned to appreciate their warm and friendly ways with the residents, their group process skills, and their interest in leading activities promoting physical and emotional health. They had learned how to turn a day room with a dozen individuals dozing or watching television into a lively interactive group.

Several of the program's graduates have already advanced to responsible jobs at nursing homes and senior centers as activity directors, program coordinators, and group leaders.

WHAT HAPPENED TO THE CLUB MEMBERS

As I mentioned above, the Club Members of the Montgomery College Adult Health and Development Program were fairly well-functioning older adults who had joined our program to improve their physical and emotional well-being—"You don't have to be sick to feel better." Some of them had recently been widowed or had suffered other personal losses among friends or family, others were living alone, all were retired, most had minor physical complaints (possibly psychosomatic), and many were lonely and bored. Some joined just for the sheer adventure of a unique experience.

There was a seemingly frail lady of eighty-two who wanted to learn to swim and did; a Chinese couple who felt isolated from the American community; several widows and widowers, many with arthritic conditions; several whose children had moved away from the area; and so on. All enjoyed the novel experience of being on a college campus at their age and the warm contacts with students and faculty.

Although our main objective was to train students for working in senior citizen facilities with older adults, the gratifying spin-off was what happened to our seniors. These people were of a generation that put value on presenting a composed facade and on not admitting to anxiety. Now they began to feel secure enough to reveal and express their emotions. For example, the exercise and relaxation techniques which seemed to have positive effects on blood pressure, sleeping patterns, and arthritis, also freed up communication and creativity. Some are working with the faculty on a new curriculum for themselves which will provide many of the learning experiences they missed during their busy years. Some have volunteered for our individual tutoring program for students who need individual attention.

Some are going to sign up for Mental Health 212X next year to help train a new batch of students. Most are going out into the community to spread the word, to tell about how much better they feel—"My back doesn't hurt anymore; I'm not so tired and depressed; my migraines have stopped"—and how much fun the experience was.

SUMMARY AND CONCLUSIONS

This story is a report of a fifteen-week exploratory course at Montgomery Community College in Montgomery County, Maryland, using group training methods to prepare students for group work with older adults. Twenty-one students, twenty-four older adults, and three faculty members from the Mental Health Associate program had gathered together to develop a training program by combining experiential T-group techniques with didactic lecture, discussion, and applied practice methods. Through this process we were able to create a learning environment in which both students and clients learn new skills and attitudes toward old age, and in which the potential of every individual is facilitated through interaction with sensitive leaders and empathic others.

> For no man can reveal to you aught but that which already
>   lies half asleep in the dawning of your knowledge.
> If he is indeed wise, he does not bid you enter the house of
>   his wisdom, but rather leads you to the threshold of your
>   own mind.   —Kahlil Gibran, *On Teaching*

This experimental course has proven successful in at least three ways: (1) our graduates are out in the field working at various facilities for the elderly, sought out by the local human services community; (2) our Senior Club members keep returning to the college for more and bringing their friends; (3) this exploratory course is now part of the regular curriculum at Montgomery Community College.

REFERENCES

Burnside, I. M. (1978), *Working with the Elderly: Group Processes and Techniques*. North Scituate, MA: Duxbury Press.
Dangott, L. R., & Kalish, R. A. (1979), *A Time to Enjoy: The Pleasures of Aging*. Englewood Cliffs, NJ: Prentice-Hall.

Gibran, K. (1965), *The Prophet*. New York: Knopf.

Leviton, D. L. (1975), Developing an adult health program model. Unpublished manuscript.

Schutz, W. C. (1960), *Firo: A Three-Dimensional Theory of Interpersonal Behavior*. New York: Holt, Rinehart & Winston.

Yalom, I. D. (1975), *The Theory and Practice of Group Psychotherapy*. New York: Basic Books.

Name index

Abraham, K., 67, 85
Aiken, L. R., 89, 91, 104
Altman, K. P., 91, 104
Altschuler, J., 10, 22
Alzheimer, A., 197
Anderson, S., 146, 148
Aparacino, 16
Arens, D. A., 134, 137
Aronson, M., 189, 196, 192, 193
Atholz, J., 9, 22
Atkinson, S., 18, 13, 27

Bach–Peterson, J., 190, 196
Baker, F. M., 7, 22
Barnes, E. K., 15, 22
Barnes, G., 139, 148
Barnes, R. F., 196
Barron, E., 10, 22
Beck, A. T., 4, 15, 22
Beethoven, Ludwig von, 220
Benaim, S., 10, 22
Bennett, R., 4, 25
Berezin, M. A., 13, 22, 67, 85
Berger, L. F., 15, 22, 68, 85, 108, 119
Berger, M. M., 15, 22, 68, 85, 108, 119
Berkman, B., 3, 22
Berland, D. I., 6, 7, 22, 114, 117, 119, 154, 162, 177, 179, 180, 186
Betcher, R. W., 154, 163
Beverly, D., 161, 163
Bienenfeld, D., 178, 186
Birren, J. E., 122, 130
Blackman, D. K., 122, 130
Blake, W., 231
Blank, L., 43, 54
Blank, M. D., 22

Blank, M. L., 9, 22
Blau, D., 13, 22
Blazer, D. G., 177, 178, 179, 180, 186
Blivise, M. D., 15, 21, 26
Bloor, M. J., 179, 182, 186
Blos, P., 85
Blum, J., 67, 80, 85
Blum, J. E., 3, 23
Blumenthal, J., 13, 25
Boas, F., 237, 244
Bolton, C. R., 10, 23
Boriello, J. F., 152, 163
Bowlby, J., 36
Breckenridge, J., 15, 28
Bremer, J., 4, 9, 16, 26
Bressler–Feiner, M., 68, 85
Brody, E. M., 90, 91, 104
Brok, A. J., 64, 65, 66, 165, 175
Buchanan, D. R., 91, 104
Burnside, I. M., 3, 18, 23, 68, 85, 86, 133, 137, 165, 174, 271, 272, 278
Busse, E. W., 177, 178, 179, 180, 186
Bussee, E., 68, 86
Butler, R. N., 8, 23, 44, 46, 48, 54, 55, 122–123, 130, 137, 136, 156, 161, 163, 178, 179, 186, 215, 219, 220

Cacciola, E. J., 23
Campbell, R., 9, 27
Caplow–Lindner, E., 233, 242
Carriere, L., 122, 130
Carroll, P. J., 20, 23
Cath, S. H., 67, 85, 212, 220
Chace, M., 234, 238, 242
Chekhov, A. P., 264
Chien, C. P., 10, 20, 23

281

Subject Index